Understanding Learning and Related Disabilities: Inconvenient Brains

Children with developmental disabilities inhabit a gray zone: they live and learn under normal conditions in some aspects of their lives, while their "inconvenient brains" present a range of challenges in other school and life contexts. Dr. Martha Bridge Denckla provides parents and educators with general knowledge, research findings, and practical recommendations about a variety of these developmental conditions, including dyslexia, dyscalculia, ADHD, autism spectrum disorder, problems with motor coordination, and executive dysfunction. Inspired by her efforts to explain these conditions to parents over 45 years of clinical practice, she provides a science-based understanding of the issues in an accessible format. She uses the science of cognitive and behavioral neurology to help readers understand how the interrelationships of brain, environment, and behavior produce these developmental disorders, and to provide a basis for parenting and education programs based upon understanding how variations in brain development should guide plans for *what* is taught *when* to *whom*. Such developmentally appropriate, evidence-based, differentiated instruction within general education can diminish the demand for separate special education, and will thus serve all kinds of brains, whether "typical" or "inconvenient."

Martha Bridge Denckla, M.D., is an honors graduate of Harvard Medical School who trained in Cognitive/Behavioral Neurology with Norman Geschwind. She has worked in hospitals affiliated with Columbia and Harvard Universities before the longest span of her career at the Kennedy Krieger Institute/Johns Hopkins. For half a century she has devoted clinical and research efforts to developmental learning disabilities and related school problems, contributing to more than 200 publications. Dr. Denckla has taught educators as well as those with neurological backgrounds.

Understanding Learning and Related Disabilities: Inconvenient Brains

Martha Bridge Denckla

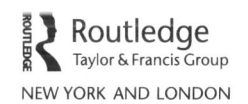

Routledge
Taylor & Francis Group
NEW YORK AND LONDON

First published 2019
by Routledge
711 Third Avenue, New York, NY 10017

and by Routledge
2 Park Square, Milton Park, Abingdon, Oxon, OX14 4RN

Routledge is an imprint of the Taylor & Francis Group, an informa business

© 2019 Taylor & Francis

The right of Martha Bridge Denckla to be identified as author of this work has been asserted by her in accordance with sections 77 and 78 of the Copyright, Designs and Patents Act 1988.

All rights reserved. No part of this book may be reprinted or reproduced or utilized in any form or by any electronic, mechanical, or other means, now known or hereafter invented, including photocopying and recording, or in any information storage or retrieval system, without permission in writing from the publishers.

Trademark notice: Product or corporate names may be trademarks or registered trademarks, and are used only for identification and explanation without intent to infringe.

Library of Congress Cataloging-in-Publication Data
Names: Denckla, Martha Bridge, author.
Title: Understanding learning and related disabilities : inconvenient brains / Martha Bridge Denckla.
Description: New York, NY : Routledge, 2019. | Includes bibliographical references and index. |
Identifiers: LCCN 2018031830 (print) | LCCN 2018034798 (ebook) | ISBN 9780429425981 (master) | ISBN 9780429759642 (pdf) | ISBN 9780429759635 (epub) | ISBN 9780429759628 (mobi) | ISBN 9781138387881 (hbk : alk. paper) | ISBN 9781138387898 (pbk : alk. paper) | ISBN 9780429425981 (ebk)
Subjects: LCSH: Learning disabilities | Children with mental disabilities. | School children.
Classification: LCC RJ506.L4 (ebook) | LCC RJ506.L4 D46 2019 (print) | DDC 618.92/85889–dc23
LC record available at https://lccn.loc.gov/2018031830

ISBN: 978-1-138-38788-1 (hbk)
ISBN: 978-1-138-38789-8 (pbk)
ISBN: 978-0-429-42598-1 (ebk)

Typeset in Utopia
by Wearset Ltd, Boldon, Tyne and Wear

This book, inspired by the questions of families and educators, is dedicated to those who have made the answers possible: the children who participated in my research, the children who visited my clinic, and my own three sons, three granddaughters, and grandson.

Contents

About the Author *ix*
Acknowledgments *x*

1 Introduction *1*

2 Brain Development Relevant to "Inconveniences" *9*

3 Promoters and Enhancers of Learning and Development *17*

4 Specific Language Impairments *23*

5 Motor Coordination Factors Contributing to School Problems *32*

6 Executive Function *43*

7 Autistic Spectrum Disorder (ASD) *54*

8 Attention Deficit Hyperactivity Disorder (ADHD) *69*

9 Dyslexia *83*

10 Math and Miscellaneous Learning Disabilities *94*

11 Neuromythology *104*

12 An Inconvenient Brain in the Context of Changes in Educational Environments *113*

References *122*

Index *125*

About the Author

An honors graduate of Bryn Mawr College and Harvard Medical School who trained in Cognitive/Behavioral Neurology with Norman Geschwind, Dr. Martha Bridge Denckla has worked in hospitals affiliated with Columbia, Harvard, and Johns Hopkins Universities. For nearly half a century she has devoted clinical and research efforts to developmental learning disabilities and related school problems, contributing to more than 200 publications (journal articles and book chapters). Recently she has been teaching educators based on accumulated evidence and experience.

Her two early and still currently used direct assessment innovations are the Rapid Automatized Naming Test (RAN) for Dyslexia and the Physical and Neurological Examination for Subtle Signs (PANESS) for Attention Deficit Hyperactivity Disorder (ADHD) and other conditions involving motor development. For the past quarter-century, her focus has been on executive function as a crucial element in many learning disabilities and school problems, overlapping ADHD. During these same years at Kennedy Krieger Institute at Johns Hopkins, collaboration with the Neuroimaging Center allowed her research to connect behavior to anatomical and functional magnetic resonance imaging and to investigate the impact of genes on the causes of "inconvenient brains." Dr. Bridge Denckla has added experience from raising three sons and advising on education of four grandchildren (three girls and one boy).

Acknowledgments

I give grateful acknowledgment to those who trained me (Norman Geschwind in Cognitive/Behavioral Neurology, Edith Kaplan and Rita G. Rudel in Neuropsychology); those who welcomed me into Child Neurology (Sidney Carter, Isabelle Rapin); those under whose broader leadership I was encouraged and facilitated (Lewis P. Rowland, Charles Barlow, Samuel Drage, Hugo Moser, and Gary Goldstein); those leaders in Neuropsychology who have done me the honor of working with me (Rita G. Rudel, Jane Holmes Bernstein, Deborah Waber, Lynn Speedie, and Mark Mahone); everyone connected with Kennedy Krieger Institute, especially Michael Batza for my endowed Professorship there); the educators who have widened my perspective (Carol Gross, Mary Ellen Lewis, Mariale Hardiman, and Nancy Grasmick); and all the families who have attended my clinic or participated in my research projects.

The production of this book was made possible by Garage Band (narrative vocal setting) and Rose Levine, who transcribed what I dictated.

1

Introduction

Who am I? I am a recently retired academic neurologist, which means a person who has always had a position at an institution at which research, teaching, and patient care are requirements. I am a Professor Emerita from the Department of Neurology at the Kennedy Krieger Institute, part of Johns Hopkins University School of Medicine in Baltimore, Maryland. My training took place mostly in Boston, where I attended Harvard Medical School, trained in internal medicine at the Beth Israel Hospital affiliated with Harvard Medical School, and then trained in neurology at Boston Veterans Administration Hospital, with a famous neurologist, Norman Geschwind, who revived the field of the cognitive and behavioral subspecialty of neurology. I trained in neurology (one year of which was at Georgetown University Medical Center in the District of Columbia) and (in Boston) an added year of fellowship that was devoted to cognitive and behavioral neurology; this is the subspecialty of neurology that involves the overlap with psychology and to some extent with psychiatry. (Informational note: everyone who becomes a specialist in neurology actually passes the examination of the American Board of Psychiatry and Neurology, with [N] specified after the certification. Neurologists are a minority group, which is reflected in our relatively small influence on the *Diagnostic and Statistical Manual.*)

The field of neuropsychology, which means psychology that refers its assessment data back to the brain as the basis of behavior, was in its infancy when I trained in neurology; and indeed there is tremendous overlap between the careers of a cognitive/behavioral neurologist and a neuropsychologist. (I am a past president of the Cognitive/Behavioral Neurology Society and also a past president of the International Neuropsychology Society.)

After I was trained and went to my first position in New York in the Neurology department (with a secondary appointment in the Psychiatry department) at Columbia College of Physicians and Surgeons, I was asked by Dr. Sidney Carter to spend part of my time attending the Child Neurology Clinic. Since I had trained exclusively with adult patients, and my knowledge was about acquired rather than developmental conditions, I was somewhat taken aback by this invitation, but I did start to go every single week to the Child Neurology Clinic, in which Dr. Sidney Carter asked me to see every child whose reason for referral to the clinic is either "not talking as expected" or "not learning how to read as expected." For a number of years, I continued to work in that clinic and also to participate in doing neurological exams included in a large study that was going on in many cities in this country; this was a multisite study of over 50,000 pregnancies and their outcomes, children followed to age eight years. I was there for the seven- and eight-year-old neurological exams, so that was another way in which half of my time became distributed towards children rather than towards adults.

I continued to do consultations on adult patients who had sustained strokes or head trauma resulting in "aphasia" (meaning a loss of language capabilities) and other related cognitive deficits; my first publication, co-authored while I was a fellow, was on the subject of "dyscalculia" (loss of ability to do calculations mathematically). Then came the moment when my career veered sharply to the pediatric side; I applied for research funding with applications involving adults, aphasia, or other cognitive deficits after strokes, and I also applied for research funding concerning "dyslexia" (specific developmental reading disorder) in children. What followed was an example of "Sutton's Law"; namely, I received approved funding for work on children with dyslexia but did not succeed in obtaining funding concerning adults who had suffered brain damage due to strokes resulting in cognitive deficits.

Then I teamed up with a neuropsychologist who had been working on those children who were in those days referred to rather bluntly as "brain-damaged." This was Rita G. Rudel, Ph.D., who really gave me my "on the job training" in conducting research. Prior to working with Dr. Rudel, my own publications had been single or multiple case reports about patients; these had not really become sophisticated, well-designed research projects involving groups of children comparisons. With Dr. Rudel, I embarked on a series of studies of children with reading problems, and we contributed to a wave of research publications that emphasized the *language* basis for difficulty in learning how to read (as opposed to the visual emphasis that still prevailed on the basis of earlier concepts, when nineteenth-century accounts of reading difficulty had used such terminology as "congenital word blindness"). At this time, encouraged by Dr. Rudel, I leaned heavily upon my neurological background to embark upon studies of children's motor coordination development, at first as a rather general tool to implicate the brain in a clinical sense when we were in those days asked about the diagnosis, "minimal brain dysfunction." This was later refined, again with Dr. Rudel, to be used as a discriminative tool when attempting to understand "hyperactive boys" compared to their typically developing peers. (See the chapter that discusses Attention Deficit Hyperactivity Disorder.) Besides the motor coordination data collected and used in research during those early years, the major achievement of my collaboration with Dr. Rudel was the creation of a test called the Rapid Automatized Naming Test, which I designed based upon classical neurological training. (In the literature about loss of reading ability after strokes, my own great teacher Norman Geschwind described color naming difficulties associated with "pure alexia without agraphia.") That Rapid Automatized Naming Test has gone through two generations of further research elaboration and application by educational researchers and neuropsychologists, has been published for general use, and stands as one of my contributions to the understanding of reading. (I think of this as an example of "beginner's luck.") Once I had begun to see pediatric patients clinically and engaged in research concerning children's developmental disorders, I gradually ceased to have time to consult and teach on any but a handful of very dramatic cases in adults.

The subsequent positions I have held and during which time I have continued to work in research and do clinical work concerning children with developmental disabilities of the type we refer to as "high prevalence, low severity" (what I call "inconvenient brains") have been during a return to Boston Children's Hospital affiliated with Harvard Medical School and in the Developmental

Neurology Branch of the National Institutes of Health, within which what was then called NINDS, in Bethesda, Maryland.

For the past 30 years, I have been a Professor of Neurology, Pediatrics, and Psychiatry at an ideal place to pursue these strands of research and clinical work, the Kennedy Krieger Institute, an institute devoted to children's brain issues, which is affiliated with the Johns Hopkins University School of Medicine in Baltimore, Maryland. This ideal position fostered my continuation of research that leaned heavily on what I had learned clinically and evidence gathered from my research during that decade in my first position at Columbia's Neurological Institute.

For the past 10 years of the 30 years of my happy work life at the Kennedy Krieger Institute, I became involved with the Neuroeducation Initiative started by Dr. Mariale Hardiman at the Johns Hopkins University School of Education. For five years I taught in a masters' certificate program at the School of Education in a program designed with Dr. Hardiman, by my co-teacher Dr. Mary Ellen Lewis, M.D., Ed.D., a course entitled "Mind, Brain, and Learning." After financial difficulties there resulted in my departure from that program, I was fortunate to be a participant at Kennedy Krieger Institute in another opportunity to teach educators, this time educators who have been classroom teachers and are aiming to move up into more supervisory positions. This was created by the involvement at Kennedy Krieger Institute of Dr. Nancy Grasmick, who had been for 30 years the Superintendent of Education for the entire State of Maryland. Dr. Grasmick, Dr. Goldstein, and Dr. Mark Mahone created the Center for Innovation and Leadership in Special Education, where three or four fellows were selected each year for a full time rigorous education; I was extremely proud and delighted to participate as a faculty member in this Center.

Most of this book is based upon clinical "feedback" sessions of explanation, interpretation, and advice to parents of youngsters whom I evaluated, plus sessions sometimes with adolescents themselves, and upon the ten years of lectures to educators. Questions asked by some of these clinic attenders and educators inspired some of the more colloquial explanations I have used; but I have also used some formal terminology from neurology or related sciences when I think it is necessary for clarity.

Why am I writing this book? At first, the reason for writing this book was in response to parents whose children I had evaluated in my clinic for their school problems. I would hold 90-minute explanatory and advisory sessions with parents one week after the evaluation of their children had taken place. Some parents brought tape recorders (or more recently their smart phones) to record my explanations, but some of them would say to me, "Have you written this down somewhere so I could review it and share it with other family members or friends who have children with similar problems?"

For many years my clinic was held only one day each week and I was doing research for much of the rest of my working time, so I would smile and say that I was too much involved in writing research grant proposals or the resulting funded research publications. As I began to teach educators, they too asked whether the lecture I had just given them, PowerPoints and all, could be found in written form for them to be able to refer back to or share. It was only during the past few years of my career when my research involvement had decreased that I myself began to feel the need to write down these explanations, interpretations, and advice for parents, as well as for any teachers who might be as interested as were those whom I had been teaching either at the School of Education or the Kennedy Krieger Institute.

Thus, I decided to write a book in the first person, just as if I were talking with parents. For decades, I did this in conferences in clinic; I gave parents detailed descriptions of what I had seen in their children, followed by explanations of what the data implied. I presented to parents what evidence existed for a certain way of understanding or viewing the problem with which they and the child were coping. Finally, I tried to guide them towards sensible interventions and away from "alternatives" that over the decades came and went as fads, discredited by researchers but revived because each new generation of parents would be susceptible to superficial plausibility of what I call the "neuromythology." (Revived but discredited claims are accessible and amplified by the Internet. Speculative explanations of brain-based problems and of quick solutions or easy answers to their children's problems still proliferate.)

Over the past decade there emerged a larger purpose in my writing this book; for two decades there had been changes in our system of education, starting with the concept of "inclusion" in regular classes of the majority of the kind of children with "inconvenient brains" whose problems I have focused upon. I had begun to realize that an understanding of these unusual and substantial minorities of students, as well as an understanding of all of the variations of *typical* development in the school years K-12, had failed to be taken into account in educational policies and "reforms." I felt the need to write about my clinic attenders within the larger context of K-12 education for all students, both typical or those with "inconvenient brains." Both these somewhat different learners seen in my clinic and all students deserve to be taught in an educational system that is based upon and takes account of evidence-based developmental science, derived from at least three disciplines, neurology, psychiatry, and psychology, with a background of sociology; we know how much the environment influences everything about the child, the environment starting with epigenetic influences that start in the womb during the mother's pregnancy. My motivation for writing this book has expanded; I now want to use the topic of "the inconvenient brain" to introduce people to many kinds of "neurodiversity" (meaning variations in brains, either in developmental timetable or in lifelong brain architecture or both) that exist and should be served in the educational landscape, truly accepting universal design for learning as a philosophy and a program.

It is my hope that not only will the book be useful to parents and other relatives or caregivers of children with "inconvenient brains" and to teachers of these children, but will be useful to a wider group (practically everybody) who is concerned with the education of our society's children and adolescents.

When I first set out to write this book I was going to call it "The Optimistic Fatalist," so I suppose I should end this Introduction by explaining what I meant by that and why I changed to the subtitle "Inconvenient Brains." What I meant by "The Optimistic Fatalist" was that I was "fatalistic" about the fact that we can do very little about the fundamental architecture or timetable of development of the brain, but that I am cheerfully "optimistic" about how we can optimize everything at home, in school, and in the larger community in order to allow that brain to be molded, accommodated, and individually educated to live up to its best potential. That potential does not always allow the possessor of the "inconvenient brain" to live up to what others would prefer him or her to become across the lifespan or to meet a rigid timetable of academic achievement, so that I advocate a more individualized orientation to attaining a good life; the "inconvenient brain" itself may be quite different from what would succeed comfortably in school achievement or fulfill the dreams of parents, in much the same way that a parent cannot plan to raise an athlete or a musician. The child's brain is not a *tabula rasa* to be entirely "written upon" with the scripts of family and society, but given its own characteristics, both in rate of development and in architecture, it can be "optimized."

Now I turn to explaining how I arrived at "Inconvenient Brains." I polled audiences for this title as compared with the title "The Optimistic Fatalist" at every event at which I could pass out slips of paper to parents and teachers; the overwhelming vote was in favor of "Inconvenient Brains."

Upon receiving the winning results for "Inconvenient Brains," I realized how much I myself liked it, because I really do not like the term "disabilities" or "disorders" applied to the problems faced by the youngsters to whom I have devoted my clinical and research career for over 40 years. To me these youngsters have *different* brains in terms of either the developmental timetable or the architectural variations that are permanent in their brains; their brains are "inconvenient" for schooling and, less commonly, for certain societal demands, but really do not in my mind demand to be called "disabled" or "disordered." I've had to explain for years in my clinic that for the purposes of qualifying for services, such terminology as "disability" or "disorder" had to be employed as the "bottom line" of my report, adorned with some number that came out of an official document like the DSM-5 or from the list of special education codes used by systems of education; but that all of the research, all of the reading I had been able to engage in, and my own clinical experience over the decades had led me to this other position, best expressed by the term "inconvenient brain."

Finally, I would hope that readers will not simply read one chapter that seems to pertain to a diagnosis or a youngster of interest to them but will read most of the chapters, especially those that cover more general information about important brain systems and their developmental trajectories (motor, language, executive function) and the chapters on "Neuromythology" (the avoidance of unsubstantiated explanations and their linked therapies) and "Promotors and Enhancers" (making the case for the benefits of sleep, play, foreign languages, and music).

My final chapter does venture into policy, but is nonpartisan in its arguments. Advocacy for "my kids," the ones with the "inconvenient brains," is impossible without advocacy for evidence-based, high quality public education for all.

2

Brain Development Relevant to "Inconveniences"

This chapter will not attempt to be comprehensive in discussing brain development, but is rather an overview that will focus more specifically on the development of those parts of the brain relevant to education and more susceptible to the kinds of variations in architecture or in timetable of development that are involved in an "inconvenient brain."

Prenatally, by six to seven months out of the nine months of the pregnancy, 70 percent of the brain cells have migrated from the interior of the brain where there is a germinal matrix (a sort of storehouse of cells called neurons) and are settled down in organized layers and columns of the cerebral cortex. There is a genetic blueprint for the cortical folding (the wrinkled look of the cerebral cortex) that is similar but not identical in every person. It can be said that "brains are like faces." (When I started to do research using neuroimaging and sat with colleagues trying to become reliable in relation to each other in outlining and measuring certain areas of the cerebral cortex, we faced difficulties due to the architectural variations from one brain to another.) Just as one can say that most people have the same itemized features on their faces, the arrangement of these features is highly individual, and except for identical twins is remarkably distinguishable, one person from the other. Thus, there is a general genetic blueprint for the folding or wrinkling of the cerebral cortex, but with apparently limitless individual patterns. To repeat: *brains are like faces.*

> While nature, in the form of genes, may lay down some general outlines, tendencies and limits for brain development, nurture (epigenetics, environment) does (for both better and worse) modify the final structure and function.

Neurons, the major cells of the brain, have to get where they're programmed to settle down by a process called cellular migration. The neurons migrate along pathways determined either by the long outgrowths of other neurons, what are called the axons, or are guided by another category of cells in the brain, the glia, which are not neurons but are very important in establishing the "glue" of the architecture and later on one type for elaborating the "insulation" covering the "wiring" connections so important in the complex dynamic structure of the brain. There are also certain chemicals that attract neurons to go to genetically programmed places. These biochemicals and receptors (surfaces with complicated configurations) together form a kind of neurological "GPS" for the migrating neurons that come out of the central germinal matrix of the brain and migrate towards the cerebral cortex. It is a wondrous thing that 97 percent of these neurons go correctly to where they are supposed to be and line up in the correct layers and columns, which are quite beautiful to view under a microscope.

Neurons then have to get connected. It turns out that this is a time-sensitive process. The neurons cluster together because they have certain chemical/receptor similarities. The parts of the neuron that are long outgrowths from the body of the cells are called axons. There are also smaller incoming sprouts from the cell bodies called dendrites. When an axon that is the long extension of neuron A meets the dendrites of neuron B, we call this a "synapse." This is the microscopic level of connections; under the microscope, the brain with its many axon-dendrite connections looks like a very untidy tangled underbrush of a dense foliage.

Connections are strengthened either by some of the chemicals that seem to attract these outgrowths but also by sensory and neurological stimuli. Dendritic "arborization" results from utilization of connections. Even in the womb, the fetus kicks, turns, sucks its thumb, and by its activity level increases the motor connections in the brain. Even more remarkably, the fetus hears and increases specific auditory connections. (Remarkably, researchers have been

Chapter 2 • Brain Development and "Inconveniences"

able to demonstrate that newborn babies will suck on a nipple to hear an audio recording of their own mother's voice in preference to the voice of most other persons; this is taken as evidence that the fetus has already heard the mother repeatedly, in spite of the muffled sound reaching its fluid-filled sac and the walls of the womb.) The motor and the auditory stimuli are influencing and shaping the brain's connections in the second half of pregnancy, more so towards the last 12 weeks or third trimester.

Another feature of brain development is that pruning overlaps with proliferation. In other words, although there is a proliferation of these connections, half of the cortical motor neurons actually die, because they do not make connections and therefore are pruned. The brain is subtly sculpted by the connections between neurons at those synapses that are sensitive both to internal chemical events, to the influence of earlier-developing parts of the brain upon the cerebral cortex (what I like to call brain-to-brain activation), and the activity-dependent strengthening of connections through movement or through the other senses. This process of pruning as well as proliferation continues after birth. Microscopic connections of synapses never stop proliferating throughout life when a neighborhood is active. Long connections may never develop or may be pruned after the first ten years of life if not active (as with muscles, "use it or lose it" applies to the brain connections). Bundles of long axons make up longer circuits in what is called the "white matter" of the brain; the "whiteness" is due to the *myelin* that is produced and wrapped around axons by one specialized type of glial cell.

This very important process is called myelination. Myelination refers to the wrapping of the axons in a fatty substance that serves like the insulation covering electrical wires. Myelination starts in the last two months of the pregnancy. The full-term baby is born with some of the visual pathways and the most basic motor pathways myelinated. The importance of this "insulation" (myelin) that covers the axons is that it permits speedy signal transmission. Again, before birth there are motor and sensory axons myelinated, but in the cortex these pathways are highly segregated from each other, traffic coming in (or up) and traffic going out (or down) but not integrated at the highest level, the cortex. All of the integrating connections among the basic sensory and motor association areas are myelinated over a long postnatal process that is highly relevant to our main concern in this book, these rapid connections underpinning what is seen as "readiness" to undertake the acquisition of certain skills. For each long connection, there is a range of ages at which the critical level of myelination is reached.

> For K-12 education, the most important ongoing brain development is myelination, the laying down of "insulating material" called myelin around axons, because it is essential for speedy connections.

Once the baby is born, the networks of synapses activate; by age three years, each neuron connects to up to 10,000 others. The pruning, which I described as the "use it or lose it" process, begins. Timely experiences during critical periods give the best (but not exclusive) results in sculpting these networks. The brain growth between birth and three years of age is not characterized by much in the way of new neurons but rather the enlargement and sprouting of neuronal axons and dendrites. The inputs to the cells and the synapses grow reciprocally and selectively. Age two is the time at which the proliferation of new connections outruns the process of selective pruning, which seems to correlate well with our experience of the charming but chaotic nature of two-year-olds, whose behaviors (and the brain driving them) have been described as reflecting "blooming, buzzing confusion."

Now we must introduce the subject of the difference between boys and girls. It is a little appreciated fact that from the time of "quickening" (when the mother can feel lively movement) of the 20-week fetus, to the time of puberty (which, of course, is variable person to person and generally earlier in girls than in boys) girls' brains develop 20 percent faster than do boys' brains. Since girls reach puberty within an age range that is shifted about two years earlier than the age range within which boys reach puberty, there is a chance for boys to show "catch up" and "late blooming." I am struck by the fact that a girl in kindergarten is 20 percent more mature than a boy in kindergarten; at age five, that 20 percent represents an entire year. (I myself have collected motor coordination data that illustrates this perfectly, because the girls up until the age of puberty are showing motor coordination skills in terms of speed and precision that are running a year ahead of the boys, not only getting off to a faster start but maintaining the lead until puberty.) There is another neuroatomical sex difference in mature architecture rather than timetable of development; there are multiple connections between the two hemispheres, the two sides of the brain, that are larger in women. In girls and women there is both earlier and stronger "interhemispheric integration," connectivity facilitating coordination (including "dominance" of the left) between the functions of the left and functions of the right side of the brain, more robust than in boys.

> Girls' brains develop 20 percent faster than boys' brains from mid-gestation ("quickening") till puberty, since puberty arrives on average two years earlier for girls than for boys, there is time for "late blooming" among boys.

Some facts about brain development explain some of the puzzling characteristics of our experience with children. There is the paradox that we know how much is learned before three or four years of age in terms of skills, the most dramatic being language. On the other hand, children before approximately four years of age rarely have what is called episodic autobiographical memory. The cause of this is that the hippocampus, the part of the brain in the midsection of the temporal lobe that is the gateway to learning personal episodic history and autobiographical memory, is not connected to the cortex. We can see that a great deal is learned procedurally through other systems of the brain. How we learn language is a very special case in the human being and is somewhat mysterious. Through language we can learn facts, sometimes whole stories about our infancy and early childhood; because we can learn narratives about our early years, it may appear that we remember events when in reality we can recite the stories we have been told!

Where is language usually most importantly represented in the brain? Even in left-handed people, 95 percent of them are like right-handed people; they still have most of the language circuits in the left side of the brain, although nonright-handed people may have some lingering language representation on the right side.

> Nonright-handed people, often thought of as "lefties," do have differently organized (but not necessarily differently timed) brain development; but the vast majority of them have left-hemisphere dominance for language functions. This variant of brain organization is still a mystery.

Some researchers have found that very early, before one year of age, comprehension of language is based upon vast expanses of the right side of the brain; this comprehension is going on before there is any speech, but the babbling that will be shaped into speech by reactions and feedback from those around the child, speech that is particular to their language, is based upon the left hemisphere. We don't know exactly how these language components and sides of the brain get organized, but sometime after about a year of age, comprehension seems to mostly vacate the right hemisphere and "take up residence" in the back part of the left hemisphere, in what we call the higher order posterior association area that sits at the junction of the three big sensory/perceptual systems, the crossroads of perceptions based on the senses of hearing, seeing, and touch.

The right hemisphere develops earlier in everybody, boys and girls, than does the left. Most of school activity is left brain based. The long pathways within that left hemisphere acquire a critical amount of myelin during a period of time that may normally vary from as early as three years of age to as late as ten years of age. It is the myelination of the left hemisphere's long cerebral pathways that is necessary for rapid naming, the surrogate of fluency in the reading process.

> At every stage of brain development, there is a range of the time it takes to get to that stage, and the normal variation is greatest at the 3-year-old end, growing less and less by the 33-year-old end of the trajectory.

In addition to variations in the timing of myelination, how robustly the left and right side of the brain communicate with each other may explain how children, more often boys than girls, can be "late bloomers." It is as though the right side of the brain is a kind of "trust fund" of cognitive processes that cannot serve as enhancement or compensation for whatever is primarily dependent on the left hemisphere until there is sufficient myelination of the big bundle of connections between the two sides of the brain called the *corpus callosum.*

In adolescence, hormones increase the synaptic pruning even more than has been the case earlier, and the "use it or lose it" process is even more prominent. Hormones also stir up the emotional parts of the brain, activating behaviors based on the basic biological drives. One of the prominent parts of the emotional brain, the amygdala, enlarges, more so in boys under the influence of testosterone. At the same time, the frontal lobe connections enabling modulation of the emotional brain, including the amygdala, myelinate. We appreciate that there is a delicate timing issue, such that if that frontal lobe's emotional controls cannot communicate strongly with this very high-drive emotional brain, what we see is the poorly controlled "impulsivity" of some adolescents. Also, a form of attention/self-monitoring, manifested in recognition of errors and error correction, matures in the part of the frontal lobe that is on the midline surface (the anterior *cingulate* that runs along and over the midline of that big band we call the corpus callosum). The big band of connections between the two sides of the brain continues to myelinate and to give rise to "two work stations" (by analogy to a computer network) available to the brain's user, the central executive in the frontal lobe.

> Full maturation of the connections of the brain, meaning that it is "all wired up," takes until the early fourth decade of life, between 31 and 35 years of age.

In summary, what we recognize about brain development is that the environment influences it, even in the womb. Although there are genetic programs governing basic events, the brain is changed by every experience we have and especially so, but not exclusively, in the early years. We know that certain skills are learned more easily and become automatic in the first decade of life, the best examples being speaking with the correct accent a second language and musical performance; we will return at some other point in this book to discuss these early skills as themselves enhancers of brain development. We also know that brain development is integrated, and when we speak, in order to be clear, about language developing at a certain time and the window of best opportunity or critical period for language, in reality language typically develops in a social context and is exemplary of the fact that there are brain-to-brain activations operating in the developmental process. Of course, there are optimal learning time spans that we call "critical periods," but they are not absolutely rigid. At every stage, learning is strongly influenced by emotion, but the state of knowledge about the mechanism of interaction of cognition and emotion is still in its infancy.

Equally shrouded in mystery is that most common of variations in brains, the right-handed and the nonright-handed, of whom the best recognized are the left-handed. About 10 percent of people are left-handed, but up to 30 percent are more in the gray zone of nonright-handed or with other forms of "mixed dominance." There are no known differences in brain developmental processes associated with these outward manifestations of motor control; 95 percent of the nonright-handed still have left hemisphere dominance for language. When injured in adult life, however, the nonright-handed recover language after left hemisphere damage better than do the strongly right-handed: but to deepen the mystery, strongly right-handed women also recover better than right-handed men, probably through a different mechanism. Nonright-handed children are no more likely to have learning disabilities than are the right-handed, so differently organized brains are not destined to be "inconvenient" in school. (One exception is the inconvenience experienced by the left-handed when writing left-to-right, more inconvenient when classroom writing surfaces provided are on the right side of the seat/desk combination.)

I will end this chapter by reflecting on two kinds of "inconvenient brains" each of which represents one aspect of different development. ADHD of the most common and uncomplicated type seems to be the outcome of a "timetable" variant of brain development, with a three-year lag in cortical thickness but eventually typical cortical structure. Dyslexia, on the other hand, seems to be the outcome of a permanently different architecture, the brain variant underlying the inconvenient opposite of a talent (but often associated with talents other than in language arts).

3

Promoters and Enhancers of Learning and Development

I'm not going to discuss in the chapter all of the very obvious essential factors that promote and enhance learning and development, such as shelter, food, emotional bonding, and support; but I will start by talking about one closely related factor in this general background—*sleep*.

Rather than talking about sleep deprivation and its ill effects, although I will mention that briefly later, I'm going to emphasize that sleep is a great promoter and enhancer of learning. Many publications in the last two decades have been adding to our knowledge of the important contributions to the learning process of sleep. Both of the two major phases of sleep, both the one involved in dreaming (the rapid eye movement or REM phase) and the deeper sleep that is referred to simply as slow-wave or non-REM sleep, contribute to learning each to a different type of information or skill. I won't go into all of those details, but it is very important to recognize that consolidation of learning takes place during sleep. Sleep promotes cognitive processes, not only remembering but also problem-solving and flexibility. After having slept, the well-rested brain is able to perform filtering of important as opposed to unimportant stimuli (smell, light, noise) and to prevent sensory overload, the sense of a chaotic or fuzzy mental state. Habitual as opposed to adaptive behaviors take over the day in the absence of adequate sleep. The connectivity between the emotional brain and the frontal lobe (amygdala and medial prefrontal cortex) is enhanced by sleep. Even motor processes such as proper articulation of speech are enhanced by adequate sleep. Many of us have had the experience of being able to solve a problem after a good night's sleep, after having been stymied by the problem during the previous evening.

During sleep itself, consolidation of learning takes place, as has been illustrated by a variety of experiments in both animals and human beings. In rodents, in which direct brain recordings can be made during sleep, running mazes seems to be rehearsed during sleep. In humans, REM states of sleep seem to consolidate spatial and context-dependent learning (not directly documented by direct brain recordings but by post-sleep behavioral data).

The most well-documented and well-publicized consequence of sleep deprivation has arisen from research on the shift in circadian rhythms in teenagers, making it developmentally inappropriate and maladaptive for teenagers to have to start perhaps middle school and certainly high school early in the morning, since the typical teenage biological "clock" (what is set by their circadian rhythm) is set in such a way that they prefer to stay up until midnight and sleep until at least 7:00 a.m.! (Even better would be till 8:30 a.m.) It is a prime example of the findings of neuroscience being ignored by the official educational or government bureaucracy that in only a handful of states in this country have starting times for high school been shifted towards later hours, allowing for the best timing of adequate sleep to be possible for adolescents. (Of course, the school systems or supervisory governments argue that there are issues of safety, greater difficulty, or inconvenience in running buses for the older students at the later hours and the more numerous and local ones for the younger students earlier; this is a case in which what is biologically better for a group of students seems to take a "back seat" to logistics and economics.)

The next universal factor that enhances and promotes learning and development is that of *play*. Why do we and many animals like to play? As a matter of fact, play is a mammalian (and some avian) constant, another of those highly conserved behavioral patterns like number sense seen in "subitizing." Play seems to be important for social and communication development, seriously contributory to aspects of survival, like choosing a mate and avoiding fatal conflict. Play seems to be how social animals learn the rules of being members of relationships and groups. It sounds like an oxymoron, because play seems so "free," but we learn rules of interaction by being playful! In playing, young children learn what other human beings think is fun and what is not fun, start to build up empathy when playmates are injured, and also how to receive and give effective nonverbal or vocal signals. Play allows young children to learn what their limits are and to differentiate which playmates have which preferences and which are shared preferences. All highly social animals seem to have play deeply embedded in their brains. Play seems to be crucial to how all social animals learn beyond that which is instinctual and even how to implement what is instinctual (such as mating). Even kittens, part of that not terribly social species, cats, are dependent upon others' social cues in order to avoid dangerous interactions. Such kittens, if deprived of opportunities to play with other kittens, are still able to hunt; but they may get into fights that kill them more readily than those who have learned how to play and learned the signals that prevent unnecessary or dangerous aggression. At younger ages and in group settings, human beings need to play in order to similarly avoid unnecessary or dangerous aggression and to learn how to negotiate with others, how to win friends and influence others. Those who look like they might be at risk for ADHD who are given extra play time (with adult supervision, of course, provided in an unobtrusive way) seem to show marked improvement in modifying their risky behaviors, as reported by parents and teachers. Connections between the emotional brain and the frontal cortex are enhanced by play. This is why play should be a universal and central part of education for children in the age group three to six years of age. Not only are young children ready and eager to play, but they *need* it as a scaffolding for life in communities of every size.

Then there is the enhancing factor afforded by early and real-life or true "*bilingualism.*" Bilingual brains turn out to have many advantages. Although there's no separate or enlarged area of the brain utilized in learning more than one language, it is a remarkable fact that the connectivity and the elaboration of the connections among neurons within the language area are enhanced in persons who are truly bilingual or "polyglot" (more than two languages are spoken) such that the neural structures are engaged in complex circuits by different languages. We must recall that extensive brain resources are dedicated to language, mainly on the left side of the cerebral cortex. There is no circumscribed area we can call "the language cortex" the way we can talk about the "visual cortex" for visual processing. If you learn a tonal language like Chinese, you also use the right hemisphere to process and program the different tones. If you are a bilingual individual who speaks English and Chinese, you actually activate both hemispheres when using and responding to the tonal differences. So there's a stage in which bilinguals speaking a European language and a tonal language will shift to actually communicate between the right hemisphere discriminating between tones to interpreting in the left hemisphere the linguistically meaningful associations of the tones. Bilingual experience is a uniquely well-researched aspect of what we call "neuroplasticity," meaning that functional and physical changes in the brain are induced by the regularly performed activities of different language complexities. You also must use your frontal lobe in order to make the pragmatic shift from one language to the other. The bilingual brain becomes strengthened in terms of the actual amount of both gray matter (neurons, brain cells) and white matter (connections). The bilingual brain is more flexible, because in circumstances in which one has to shift from one language to the other, there is repeated exercise of "code-switching" that requires the involvement of the frontal lobe control over the capabilities of this highly elaborated language network.

Musical training, even if not sustained after the first decade of life, has enhancing effects. After many years of research being performed concerning trained and professional musicians, more recently neuroscientists have turned to studying young adults in terms of the impact of past musical training. Young adults, even those not actively engaged in musical activities (and listening doesn't count in what I am reporting here), with as little as one year of actual training on some kind of musical activity, playing an instrument or singing (but not just listening to music) before the age of ten, showed brain changes maintained for life; enhanced were attention to and perception of sounds, so that in all kinds of communication situations such as noisy rooms or environments (like transportation settings) auditory skills were very much better in those who had had even that brief one-year duration of musical training before puberty. The brain signals that were being measured in young adults were reliable representatives of auditory signals; key elements of the sound signals captured by the nervous system were strengthened in those who had the early active musical instruction. Music enhanced brain functional capacity to deal with the auditory-based educational system, fundamental and essential, so speech and language become beneficiaries of music education. (To repeat; this is *not* the passive "music appreciation" class, it is the instruction in skills needed to produce music.) Enhanced auditory perception extends also into a component of executive function (selective auditory attention) and auditory communication skills. In addition, because rhythmic aspects of music and their numerical representations, in counting and in the notation system, are processed in the left side of the brain, while the pitches, tones, and keys are processed in the right side of the brain, musical activities promote and enhance interhemispheric integration. Since this collaboration between the two sides of the brain at the cortical level is so important in mathematics, it has been suggested that musical skills prepare and enhance the brain for mathematics. (There are many anecdotes about musical mathematicians, but little solid research concerning this intriguing association.)

While there is some work similar to that for music concerning dance and other kinds of movement instruction, it is not as well developed as the work on music in terms of benefit to brain development and functional enhancement. Also sparse in research but replete with anecdotes (inviting further research) are the benefits of the visual graphic arts; emotional benefits, some mediated by rising levels of the neurotransmitter, serotonin, have been reported, with corresponding "brain waves" indicating a calming effect. As with music, producing art has a greater effect than viewing it. Quite a separate issue is whether the visual arts are useful adjuncts to traditional academic instruction, what is often referred to as "art-infused education." Of course, as I have emphasized throughout this book, all activities and learning experiences change the brain, but the issue here is whether antecedent effects, as with bilingualism or musical activity, can be demonstrated, or whether art activity woven into traditional academic curriculum has concomitant "booster" effects, could be used in compensatory strategies, or provides a positively reinforced success in the school environment that makes it easier to tolerate the fatigue and frustration some students experience in learning school skills.

This is a more general sense in which the "extracurricular activities" in schools, the arts and athletics, enhance learning and brain development; this is the sense in which the emotional life of a student provides a general background of positivity to the school experience and a more specific sense of self-confidence to the individual. Particularly for those individuals who are those we describe as having "inconvenient brains" for the traditional academic curriculum, competence or, even better, excellence in one of the arts (music, visual arts, dance, theater) or in athletics, provides evidence that the individual *has* a problem but contradicts the depressing thought that the individual *is* a problem.

Published research reports that those high school students who are classified as having learning disabilities but who are engaged and successful in what we call "extracurricular activities" benefit more from their remedial and general education courses and graduate from high school in higher numbers than do others with learning disabilities who lack these extracurricular achievements. The way I see it, these accomplishments amount to "emotional bank accounts" upon which youngsters with "inconvenient brains" can draw for the energy, motivation, and self-esteem that carry them through school and may, directly or indirectly, form the core of post-educational vocational successes.

4

Specific Language Impairments

We are so interested in language development and language impairments because most learning disabilities are language based to some extent, even if language appears adequate for life outside of school and does not rise to the level of recognized language impairment. Most language impairments that rise to the threshold of being considered within the category of specific diagnosis, called Specific Language Impairment (SLI), are brought to some kind of professional attention due to a delay in either comprehension or talking or both in the very early years of life, ideally starting with recognition and some level of intervention by no later than the age of two years and six months. Of course, hearing impairment must be ruled out or recognized as a factor, the most urgent diagnosis and intervention.

The definition of an SLI is that it is not due to a general cognitive deficit, although of course in the very early years there are not many ways to assess cognitive abilities aside from language, since language is the outstanding cognitive achievement of early development. Also, SLI is not supposed to be due to poor hearing, but the degree to which some degree of imperfect hearing contributes is not always entirely clear. Sometimes what seems "common sense" is disproven; I participated in a large study many years ago in which we went into the research absolutely convinced that multiple middle ear infections involving inflammation and fluid in the middle ear would impair hearing; and that this would be a cause of SLI. Our conviction was overturned by the data, in which it turned out that many children suffered significant numbers of ear infections, even severe enough to necessitate having tubes placed in the eardrum to drain out fluid, and yet showed no significant language delay. Also, in a far more complicated context, an SLI was not supposed to be secondary to Autistic Spectrum Disorder; but language impairment is a major part of the communication dysfunction central to most with Autistic Spectrum Disorder.

The important "take home" message for this chapter is that even minor, superficial, or residual aspects of language impairment, even when this has been remediated or has responded to intervention to the degree that no one would maintain a formal diagnosis of SLI, still remains the link to school problems. It can be stated quite emphatically that language is linked most obviously to reading and written expression, but, perhaps less appreciated, also to mathematics, which has its own language. (For example, it was demonstrated even before I was a professional that children with Down Syndrome, who generally have a particularly severe language component to their intellectual disability, benefit from language therapy involving intensive lessons on "the language of mathematics"; as a result of such intervention, these intellectually limited children make much better progress in arithmetic than would be otherwise expected from their intelligence quotients.)

> Language development and language impairment should be in the foreground of concerns about school, separate from Autistic Spectrum Disorder and contributory to the problems and the effective interventions in reading and written expression in those we say have dyslexia, which is a subtle language-based learning disorder.

We know something about the brain/neurological basis of SLI, but even at the level of "localization in the brain" problems arise. The more fine-grained knowledge is still lacking or contradictory across different studies. We know quite certainly that the left side of the brain and the language systems in that left side of the brain are implicated in SLI; it has been reported in studies using magnetic resonance imaging (MRI) as varied in terms of exactly *where* within the left side of the brain the impairments might arise. In some groups there are smaller structures around the fissure that separates the temporal from the parietal lobe; in other studies, the smaller structural region is the inferior frontal area, sometimes on both sides of the brain. There are even some studies that implicate the volumes of structures such as thalamus or basal ganglia, subcortical structures that connect with the cerebral cortical lobes mentioned above. Remarkably, except for the localization to the left hemisphere, more focal brain correlates of the different language impairments has not been consistent.

Language is assuredly an incredibly complex set of functions, so that its development still remains a fascinating subject of study, with many details not yet known to us. Competency in language first involves the analysis of speech sounds that are rapidly changing and that encode and store a great deal of multilayered information. For most infants, the drive to pay attention and to select certain speech sounds arises in the social-emotional interaction with caregivers.

The chapter on dyslexia refers to a way of visualizing language as an "iceberg." At the very broad base of the "iceberg,"

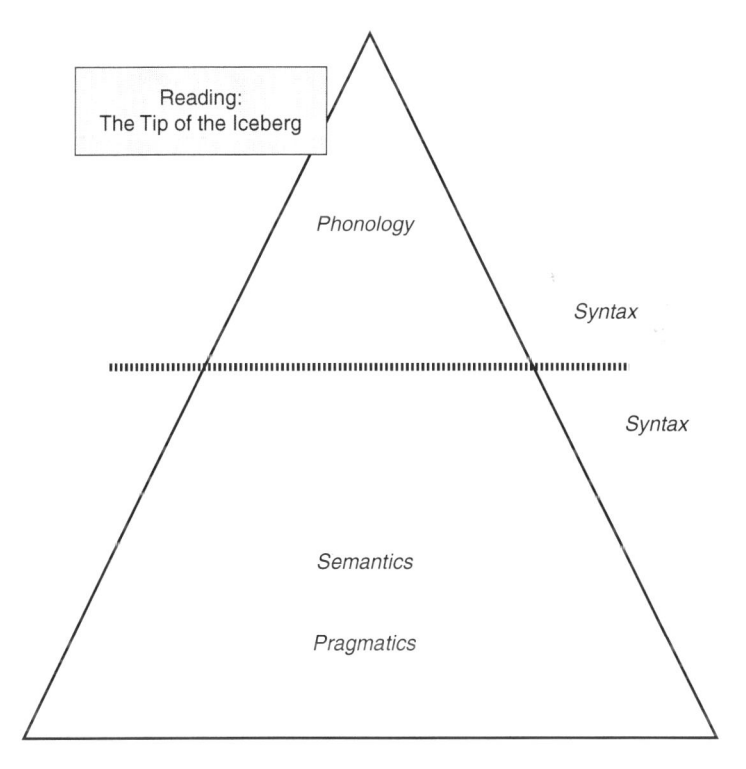

Figure 4.1 The levels of language, from most communicative to most speech specific.

underneath the surface of the water, are the pragmatics, which means the practical, everyday, interpersonal context of communication. At the next level of the "iceberg," but still under the surface of the water, are the "semantics," which means the meaningful associations of the speech sounds, dependent upon that big, distinctively human brain region that wraps around the back of the fissure between temporal and parietal lobes, called the "temporal-parietal" higher order association area. What exactly happens in order for some speech sounds to be able to be both understood as or spoken as representations of all the outside world and the inner world of feelings that we experience with all our senses is one of the great challenging mysteries of neuroscience and one of the "crowning glories" of human evolution.

One of the interesting things about speech sounds, described in the chapter on dyslexia as well as here, is that they are not strictly "auditory" information; a scientific recording called an acoustic spectrogram cannot actually pick up an isolated speech sound but can only pick up blends between consonants and vowels. In fact, I have been thinking of the unit of speech sound, the formal name being a "phoneme," as made up of an auditory perception linked to a mouth position, much as the chemical formula for water is "H_2O." In other words, one of the things that is so misleading both in the study of SLI and the study of reading problems is the idea that "auditory processing" in a global sense is the root of these problems. To repeat, the unit of a speech sound or phoneme is not strictly auditory but is an amalgam of auditory perception with mouth position. It's fascinating to contemplate that babies babble spontaneously and then have their babbling shaped by the responses of those who take care of them and respond to their babbling. Babies babble producing sounds that occur in many different languages around the world; but when they do not get positive feedback in response to some of those productions, those particular "mouth gymnastics" destined to be "foreign" drop out. More than one set of speech sounds can be handled by the infant if different caregivers speak different languages.

SLI comes in different varieties. It can be strictly expressive, meaning that reception or understanding of what is said is perfectly normal. There are mixed expressive/receptive language disorders, often more severe expressive than receptive. Of course the most severe are those conditions when language received by the child's brain or language expressed out of it is equally impaired. Expressive language impairment can exist with perfectly normal *speech*! Here again, there is a tendency to think that children who have normal speech, who articulate all the speech sounds and thus do not need to go to a "speech therapist," cannot possibly have an expressive language disorder. They may have a very good brain circuit for learning the procedures used in producing the "mouth gymnastics" that are associated with speech sounds, but they may have some weakness in connecting with the semantic level, the meaningful level of language.

One of the imaging findings common to both SLI and dyslexia is a completely symmetrical region of the temporal lobe that goes by the name of the *"planum temporale."* The interesting thing here is that in persons who are well endowed with language (and that includes the ease of acquiring reading), the left *planum temporale* is ten times the size of its "mate" on the other side, the right side. In research studies examining the MRIs of SLI and dyslexic groups, there tends to be seen that no temporal region, left or right, is smaller; rather, there is more equal volume of brain tissue on both the right and the left side of the brain. The reason that I issue such a severe warning about using the rather overgeneralized term "auditory processing" is because that right-sided *planum* is important for three kinds of auditory processing that are "nonverbal." These other kinds of auditory processing are 1) understanding the emotional message conveyed or connoted by the rise and fall of the voice, 2) discriminating between different environmental sounds (doorbell, phone ringing, dog barking), and 3) discriminating between musical pitches, what we think of as musical talent, "an ear for music." The left side in the typically developed language-competent person has the "lion's share" of the processing space on the left side, which is the brain region in which auditory processing is devoted to speech sounds and has nothing to do with tone of voice, environmental noises, or musical pitch (although rhythm may involve the left side as well).

Getting back to what is actually seen as deficient in SLI, there seems to be some kind of limited processing capacity or processing speed with respect to speech sounds. This limited capacity in many cases extends to working memory for words and for phonemes, both the meaningful and the strictly "speech sound" components of language. The idea that slow speech sound processing is the underlying deficit is sometimes incorporated into a more general theory that all auditory processing, not limited to speech sounds, is slow and is the basis of SLI, but the bulk of evidence is that the system on the left side, the dedicated speech sound system, is usually the one that is inadequate or at least less well endowed.

If one looks at the lifespan of those with SLI, one wonders how purely "specific" is the impact of this "inconvenient brain," aside from the fact that there is (when first diagnosed) a robust nonverbal IQ. (By definition, to be included as qualifying for SLI, nonverbal cognition must be within normal limits.) There is a curious fact that the nonverbal IQ, at least in the forms we are capable of assessing it, seems to decline with age in association with SLI, more spectacularly in girls than in boys. Most with SLI will go on to show dyslexia, although it is remarkable and perhaps a clue as to their subtype of SLI, that one-third of these children do fine in the acquisition of the basic decoding skills level of reading. (I suspect, although I have no evidence to confirm this, that those whose speech articulation is spared from their expressive language impairment are those who can master phonics.) All with SLI have difficulty with reading *comprehension* beyond the level of basic decoding. This group contributes to the deviation from "the simple view of reading," that comprehension follows decoding as night follows day.

The largest group of those screened and referred for SLI have a mixed expressive/receptive disorder, but often the expressive is the more severe part of the mixture. Many with SLI also have Developmental (Motor) Coordination Disorder (D(M)CD) and Attention Deficit Hyperactivity Disorder (ADHD). Thus, the word "specific" captured in the name SLI is meaningful only relative to a measurement of nonverbal cognitive ability.

As has been suggested already, the academic course of those with SLI is that the reading comprehension stage of language arts learning is a difficult one. Mastering written expression is extremely difficult. Even when assessment for oral language seems to yield results within normal limits, more subtle language deficiencies show up in reading comprehension, which is often the lagging indicator of a real "recovery." This is even when the basic reading skills have been either remarkably normal, as is the case in about a third of those with SLI, but also after an excellent response to the remediation of the basic reading skills in the other two-thirds. (I have mused that we need a category of "academic language impairment," because what is "good enough for daily life is not good enough for school.")

Most identified with SLI are "late talkers" and if not provided with interventions will acquire their language skills very slowly, really lagging behind the language accomplishments of their peers. Often grammar, in both reception and expression, is identified as the most impaired feature of their language assessment; but unfortunately, word-finding difficulty, best tested in the most academically relevant way (naming pictures), is often not well appreciated. In the academic course of SLI, this word-finding difficulty, sometimes referred to as "word retrieval" difficulty, may persist long after the student is dismissed from services intervening to improve language. Partly this is due to the fact that new words are almost daily being introduced in the school setting, demanding vocabulary retention and retrieval far beyond what is required in daily life.

In summary, there are many language processes that, when not strong enough to make school comfortable, need extra support if we expect adequate progress in school. We have mentioned the phonological (speech sound) processes and the vocabulary processes linked to basic reading and reading comprehension, but there are also large contributions of language to arithmetic and more complex mathematics, which were mentioned in the context of intellectual disability but are still true in the context of specific language SLI. There is no school subject at any level that is not heavily dependent on a large repertoire of language processes. Grammatical complexity is characteristic of "word problems" in mathematics and algebra may be described as "naked syntax," relationships of "x" and "y" manipulated without numbers specified until the end of the problem.

Let's look at the adaptive functions across the lifespan of the population with SLI. In the early years, these late talkers consistently score lower on a personal social competence scale because it is so common that responses of parents are heavily influenced by their child's ability to communicate using language. This goes on to affect socialization with peers, although it may happen somewhat later among boys than among girls. Because boys generally develop speech and expressive language somewhat later than girls (with the exception of receptive understanding of language, which is about equal) boys may be more able to socialize and communicate using their movements and actions in a nonverbal way, while even when very young girls tend to be "chatty" in social situations. A neurodevelopmental dysfunctional picture of a broader, less specific type is very frequently highlighted by the "late talking" and lagging language. Important compensatory factors are that those with SLI who are the first born and have mothers with high levels of education and income do much better than others with SLI; their language stimulation is both an epigenetic enhancer of brain development and a form of therapy.

Jumping over the elementary school age group and the enormous effects of language processes on academic achievement, when we look at adolescents, SLI groups still lag in language areas and, in general, IQ scores, both verbal and nonverbal, decline. There are social problems, now in boys as well as girls. Adolescents with SLI seen in clinic will often tell sad stories of how much trouble they have "kidding around" with their friends; they don't "process" a joke quickly enough to laugh at the appropriate time, and they have a great deal of trouble interjecting a quip or witty comment at the appropriate moment in the flow of jocular conversation. These adolescents with SLI, boys as well as girls, explain that they often remain silent because their slow processing makes their laughter or their own attempts at joking so badly timed that they seem "weird."

Adolescents with SLI often seem to show increased attentional problems even if they do not have the coexisting diagnosis of ADHD; listening to teachers explaining or lecturing in these advanced grade levels imposes such a load upon them, they lag so far behind in processing the language, that they lose focus. (I explain to them that this is like plugging into too many outlets sharing the same electrical circuit and "blowing a fuse.")

To conclude this chapter, I will not discuss language therapy, a specialized and very important kind of therapy carried out by speech/language pathologists, except to say that I think that more of it continued for many years should be provided than is currently the case. Many of the same principles guiding language therapy are discussed in the chapter on dyslexia, but the professional group providing language therapy is even more highly specialized than are educators. (Note that I emphasize language, not speech, therapy.)

There is no more pervasively important developmental difference with impact upon the "landscape" of education than SLI, even if language impairment is mild in its impact on daily life. Sadly, SLI has been eclipsed (even in the DSM-5) by emphasis on Autistic Spectrum Disorder (a more severe syndrome within which there is often language impairment) or, to a lesser extent, by dyslexia (a subtle language-based impairment).

5

Motor Coordination Factors Contributing to School Problems

This is probably the most unusual chapter to include in a book on school problems. Undoubtedly, it reflects the fact that I am a neurologist rather than a psychologist (although due to my training and research collaborations I regard myself as an "unofficial" neuropsychologist), but I do feel that there has been a lack of appreciation of the degree to which motor coordination problems, especially those involving handwriting, contribute to school problems.

First let me begin with an anecdote. About three decades ago, when one of my sons was returning from college and found himself sitting next to another college freshman also returning to the area where we lived, it was remarkable that when they exchanged names this other young man said to my son, "Oh, are you related to Dr. Martha Denckla? She saved my life." This elicited a laugh from my son, who responded to his classmate by saying that surely he was mistaken; his mother, Dr. Denckla, did not work in any emergency room or hospital and hadn't dealt with physical threats to life in many years. My son could not see how this young man could say that having been seen in my clinic resulted in "saving [his] life." The young man then explained that he had been floundering in school despite being a very good reader and quite gifted in mathematics, had become a chronic underperformer and underachiever due to the fact that he was struggling so much with his handwriting; but Dr. Denckla had provided him and his family with an understanding of his handwriting problems and had recommended accommodations to create detours or compensations for them. When these interventions were implemented, the young man continued, he began to like school and to do well, consequently being a freshman in the same excellent college attended by my son.

I tell this anecdote not to pat myself on the back (although it was pleasant to have someone convey respect for me to my teenage son), but to emphasize that in many cases struggles with handwriting create big problems for students, not the least of which is what I like to think of as aversive conditioning towards doing the work that has to be written on paper, in school but even more so to complete homework. Parents get involved in struggles over homework, and students procrastinate or find excuses to avoid doing homework, creating very difficult scenes at home more than in school. When the handwriting problems seem unexpected in relation to the good skills in the other major aspects of education, reading and mathematics, the child with poorly developed handwriting skills is often interpreted by both parents and teachers as simply "not trying" or "oppositional" because the child has declared defensively that the written work is "boring," although many complain that handwriting is uncomfortable and fatiguing.

> Motor development has direct significance for athletics and/or handwriting skill. While handwriting is neither taught nor given grades in school, handwriting difficulty and discomfort is a major source of school problems, even escalating to dislike or rejection of attendance at school.

I'm starting out with handwriting because it is probably the most important component of what is known as Developmental Coordination Disorder (DCD) that does appear in the *Diagnostic and Statistical Manual* (DSM-5). DCD is defined as a marked impairment in the development of fine, "gross," or global motor coordination and is said to affect 6 percent of school-age children. In addition, these children are characterized as developmentally impaired or delayed in motor learning and new motor skill acquisition. To a neurologist, the latter characterization is what we would call "dyspraxia." (The term "dyspraxia" is not so intimidating if one realizes its roots in words like "practical" and "practice.") In any event, the "fine motor coordination" element is very frequently expressed in the handwriting struggles of these children and is not necessarily accompanied by more general or global motor coordination difficulties, which also may have both school and home impacts.

Because of my background in behavioral and cognitive neurology, I tend to avoid the term "developmental dyspraxia" because some of the requirements for what has to be demonstrably intact in adults with acquired dyspraxia simply cannot be present in children who have difficulty with motor skills. In adults, underlying control of the muscles and movements should be intact and the skill should be available with full "real-world" stimuli, showing that some connection has been lost. Because it is unusual to be able to document in a child that basic motor control is intact, because the line between basic and skilled movement is difficult to establish developmentally, it is impossible to describe impaired acquisition as "lost." I prefer to simply say that children with DCD show motor skills learning disability and not use the term "dyspraxia." (After all, we do not use the term "dysphasia" for developmental speech/language impairment.)

As with reading, speech, and language disorders, one can take a look at handwriting and see different levels/different brain contributions that are reasons handwriting is impaired, although all of them are related to the brain's multiple overlapping motor systems. The difficulty in motor learning would obviously be at a higher order level and involves a procedural learning circuit that is very similar to the one involved in learning how to read, with a component of visual perception having to be linked to motor patterns or motor movements. Far more common, however, is the more literally motor control level of the developmental trajectory, the actual ability to receive from the highest level of the brain the signals that go to the fingers. If young children are given writing implements (usually pencils), they will show us immediately by the way they grasp the pencil whether or not they are able to receive signals for control that would go all the way down to the thumb and index finger of the preferred hand. (The middle and other fingers mainly serve as stabilizers of the posture (more about postural stability a little later) and the movement is controlled from the very tips of the first two fingers. This involves very little energy consumption and therefore can be engaged in for long periods of time comfortably, which in turn leads to more practice, which in turn leads to more rapid automatization of the motor movements involved and greater speed in the procedure. Handwriting is the best example of a skill acquired through procedural learning. Very frequently, in a sizable majority of children (boys more often than girls) there is a developmental delay in the efficient pathway being facilitated by the process of myelination (please see chapter on brain development); if immature, this allows rapid signals to get only as far as the hand, not the fingers. When one looks at a child's pencil grasp and sees that the pencil is actually grasped in what we call the web space between the base of the thumb and the base of the index finger, one sees that the movement is actually coming from the hand rather than from the ends of the fingers. This entails using a much larger set of muscles (hand rather than fingers) to move the pencil; this is slower, more energy-consuming, and can be more uncomfortable (some children say painful) than the really efficient pencil control from the ends of the fingers, thumb and index. The consequence of this proximal pencil grasp and use of hand muscles is that handwriting is a really uncomfortable chore, is not enthusiastically engaged in for the purpose of practice, and is a source of aversion to schoolwork. There are some cases in which very highly motivated and diligent children will persevere with this immature and inefficient pencil use, the hand-pushing type with the "incorrect" pencil grasp, tolerating discomfort to produce very nice writing. I urge parents and teachers not to be fooled by the *product* but to look at the *process*. It is also very common that those with the proximal, web-space-based pencil grasp are given corrective measures by

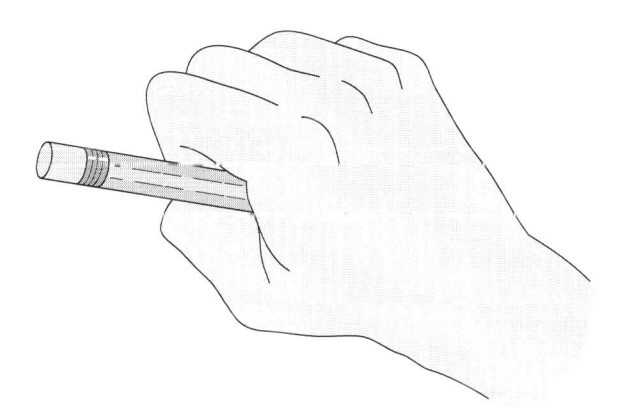

Figure 5.1 Immature pencil grasp indicating that control stops at hand muscles and persists as a maladaptive habit that is hard to break.

special education teachers or occupational therapists (fatter pencils, pencils with specially configured rubber grippers on them, and so forth). Unfortunately, these well-intentioned accommodations are not going to change the status of the brain pathway from the highest level of the brain, the frontal cerebral cortex, in the control of the proper muscles. Modification of the writing implement makes everybody feel that something is being done, but unfortunately this does not really have very much effect.

This stressful situation with the pencil control has been worsened in recent years, when academic undertakings have been pushed back at least one year and sometimes even more. This is an example of educators "killing with kindness." Children as young as three and certainly by age four in prekindergartens are encouraged to learn to write their names and to write the letters of the alphabet in print. If they are compliant and motivated children, they may do so. The level of demand is very low in those very early years and so they may simply continue to use the pencil in the inefficient way when they go into kindergarten (which is now what used to be first grade) and print words and numerals, not long afterwards being asked to write little paragraphs towards the end of the first grade (what used to be second grade). By then what has happened is the establishment of an entrenched "bad habit." This persists even after optimal development of myelination has occurred, but the most advantageous pathway is not used, due to the strength of the maladaptive habit.

Now one thing you need to recall about motor skills learning is that it is wonderful when correctly acquired and maintained even with long lapses of utilization. The best example of this is the well-known experience of going on a vacation and renting a bicycle; we are delighted to find that even though we hadn't ridden a bicycle since we were children, after a few wobbles we are able to take off and ride the bicycle, because the skill is very well conserved in our procedural brain circuits. Unfortunately, the opposite is true. Practicing a skill with less efficient muscles can become a "bad habit" that is almost impossible to break. We will talk later about how all this can be avoided and dealt with, but for the moment we simply want to state flatly that premature demands for writing, particularly printing, are ill-advised. While early introduction of printing springs from good intentions, it is, indeed, for some children, "killing with kindness." One has to look at the *natural* pencil grasp, not after one corrects it and repositions the pencil in the child's hand; but I have observed that after an interval left alone the child's grasp reverts to its natural inefficiency. In order to observe the developmental status of the child's writing control, we must be patient observers with respect to when this particular motor skill shows an "efficient final common pathway."

Then there are children who have more generalized coordination issues. These movements are often referred to as "gross motor" in contrast to handwriting being described as a leading component of "fine motor" coordination. More generalized motor coordination difficulties may result in a child being awkward even in walking and being the object of ridicule or even of exclusion by other children. Certainly when it comes to engaging in games involving running and even more so games involving using balls that have to be controlled either by the foot or by some kind of athletic tool used in the hand (baseball bat, tennis racquet, hockey stick), the child with the more generalized motor coordination impairment, what is formally called DCD, will be in bad standing with respect to peer group acceptance and consequent social-emotional development. Since sports are undertaken in school as part of either recess or as part of the physical education curriculum, these more general motor coordination problems do in fact influence whether a child likes school as well as participation in the expanded world of after-school and extracurricular activities.

The causes of DCD are not well understood but are probably similar in terms of developmental delay to the other "brain inconveniences" being discussed in this book. As I said at the outset, we who see the importance of the motor factor are in the minority in the community of professionals who deal with children's school problems; research on DCD is sparse as compared with research on reading. DCD is very commonly associated with Attention Deficit Hyperactivity Disorder (see that chapter), sometimes with Specific Language Impairment, and more narrowly in its fine motor/handwriting form with dyslexia.

As far as other fine motor coordination and motor learning issues, these could include tying shoelaces, coping with zippers and buttons of smaller size, properly brushing teeth or combing hair, and other activities of daily living. Although it is rarely emphasized to us, we see that even the use of cutlery for eating, such as the way the fork or spoon is grasped and used, or the coordination involved in using the fork and the knife to cut meat, can also be quite problematic for some children, although this is usually either ignored or easily overcome; this is because it is usually done under less pressure and less demand for either early acquisition or speed and involves less complexity, compared with what coordination and skill is demanded in school.

It is also a very curious fact that many children who have handwriting problems are quite good when it comes to drawing, painting, or doing other artistic things with their hands. They may even be good at other "fine motor" tasks like stringing beads or playing with very small items of "Lego®." Failure to appreciate that a variety of skills are included under the term "fine motor" can lead to a misinterpretation of a handwriting problem as being a question of motivation rather than a true developmental impairment or delay. ("If you can draw, why can't you write?") The fact is that handwriting is a unique "pinnacle" skill in the fine motor category and cannot be equated with even drawing or painting or any of the other "fine motor" skills. Even playing the piano may be perfectly accessible to the same child who has trouble with a pencil. The way to understand this is partly because of the muscles involved (the grasp for drawing or painting does not need to be so far out on the fingers) but also because there is a kind of abstraction about the use of a writing implement; there is no direct feedback through the sense of touch or pressure, because there are no nerve endings at the end of the writing implement, pen or pencil. The writing implement must operate either on the basis of direct visual copying in the learning phase, transitioning to letters from visual memory. To become automatic, it must be controlled from recall of visual images of letter forms and can be done (except for placement on lined paper) with the eyes closed.

Another way in which neurology might inform education would be in challenging the choice of printing to precede and sometimes completely eclipse any kind of cursive handwriting. If you look at the examinations of what is called "visual-motor coordination" as performed even in screening assessments by pediatricians, the first page starts off with asking the child to copy a circle; even an elliptical version of a circle, as long as the entire outline of the shape is closed, is accepted as a three-year-old accomplishment that is quite typical. It is only later that a child is expected to execute right angles such as in a square or, even later, diagonals such as in a triangle. The diagonals are not expected until five years of age. It would be much more generous in our expectations if we started everybody off with cursive, which is basically a sequence of continuous elliptical movements of various sizes and placements. If we return to five years as the average starting age for instruction in handwriting, we would be better advised to be teaching cursive, since the elliptical achievement has probably been in the repertoire of most children's visual-motor pathway since back when they were three years of age. While the normal distribution curve shows not all reach the diagonal "milestone" at the age of five, achievements of three-year-olds should be quite a generous comfort level for five-year-olds at the lagging end of the developmental trajectory. What we do when we demand printing is to plunge right in to the diagonals that are so much more difficult than ellipses for the control system to produce. Worse still, schools are currently demanding printing at age four years.

Of course, the other things we can do with our available technology are to forget about using any kind of handwriting and allow word-processing, what we used to call "typing." But we should not make the mistake with young children of insisting as a prerequisite "proper keyboarding skills," thereby imposing yet another hurdle and another possible source of failure. What we should do is to allow the use of the right and left index fingers, in the time-honored "hunt and peck" method that has been used by many adults (some of them great authors) who did not learn touch typing. I advise schools to allow the child to produce letters on the screen by means of this hunt-and-peck methodology. We need to de-emphasize speed in the early elementary grades; we are not preparing students for secretarial jobs. Having recommended this frequently during my clinical years, I can tell you that the child will arrive at the moment when he or she can feel capable of learning to use all of the fingers in a specified sequence, will desire the greater speed afforded by proper keyboard skills, and seek instruction at that time.

You may be wondering why I said there might be an exception for piano playing or other instrumental playing, like the very difficult use of the individual fingers on the left hand of the violin or other string instrument player; this is explained by the fact that there is combined auditory and tactile feedback for these movements. Such a pathway analysis is very important to understand neurologically; what guides the motor system in the brain makes a difference; if there is more than one guiding input from different perceptual systems, this enhances motor control and skill learning. It is an apparent paradox that a child who is musically gifted will sit down and play the piano, moving those fingers fluently and efficiently over the instrument, while at the same time laboriously, inefficiently, and uncomfortably attempting to push a pencil or pen across paper, particularly when asked to print.

Postural stability was mentioned briefly when I described the hand and fingers positions involved in handwriting, Now I must mention one other source of handwriting difficulties in children, a postural instability seen as Prechtl Choreiform Syndrome. (It was described by Dr. Prechtl, hence providing one of the rare developmental diagnoses given what we call an "eponym," the proper name of whoever described a syndrome.) The hand and fingers are involuntarily moved in irregularly timed displacements of posture, not regular like a tremor, but little jerks that are almost graceful (hence the name "choreiform," meaning "dance-like") but disruptive of the smoothness of handwriting. Seen in the clinic, those with Prechtl Choreiform Syndrome show wavy and wobbly copying of shapes, with sudden concave or convex bulges in lines; these may be compensated for by hard pressure, which may straighten out the appearance of the line but is uncomfortable, verging on painful if prolonged. Followed over years, the involuntary lapses of posture often lessen and then disappear, but this may not occur until postsecondary years. In the years till young adulthood, word-processing may be the recommended method of getting words on paper, because the movements of fingers on the keyboard do not require sustained postures. (If there are no other manifestations of DCD, the substitution of keyboarding for handwriting may be one of the rare neurologically based "cures" for a school problem.)

It may also be of interest that children who show another "eponymous" syndrome, Tourette Syndrome, the involuntary movements of which are motor and vocal tics, may show *superior* motor skills. (This is true only if there is no coexisting ADHD, just Tourette Syndrome.)

Now, turning to the more athletic and daily living parts of DCD, I would make a very firm recommendation that team sports be set aside and other individual athletic pursuits substituted. These include swimming, fencing (for eight years and over), climbing, gymnastics, ice skating, and table tennis (less demanding of running than regular tennis). In other words, individual skills rather than team sports are likely to be sources of success and social-emotional gratification for children who are poorly coordinated. Partly this is because they can learn the skills at their own individual pace, with repetitions if necessary, without the embarrassment of constantly being the one who "lets the other members of the team down," and with a sense of getting positive feedback even for small incremental improvements.

The controversial role of occupational therapy is controversial only with respect to which "school" of occupational therapy we are talking about. There are some occupational therapists who really adhere to the traditional view of occupational therapy as patiently training the child in his or her "occupations." Examples would be teaching the child how to ride a bicycle, teaching the child how to jump rope, teaching the child how to run more efficiently. With the other kind of occupational therapy, which is based on a theoretical concept that one has to intervene with exercises targeting some fundamental level of the nervous system, the guiding principle is to strive to build brain circuits serving prerequisite skills; this kind of occupational therapy does not deal directly with actual skills (the child's occupations). This more controversial form of occupational therapy is accepted as standard and is prevalent in certain parts of our country. I will return to discussing this in the chapter where I discuss popular, plausible, but largely unsubstantiated methods of treatment.

In conclusion, there are direct life impacts of DCD. In some instances, it is best to reduce demands, to alter expectations, and just wait until those maturing at the very most lagging end of the developmental trajectory have caught up to meeting the demands for the skills. I recommend that we wait and observe the child before making demands for a given skill, rather than having a fixed timetable of exactly when each motor skill is expected and therefore demanded of the child. What I am advocating is therefore a concept of "motor readiness" akin to that of "reading readiness." (Unfortunately, nowadays the entire concept of "readiness" has somehow been set aside.)

Besides the direct significance of either fine or more global DCD, there is also indirect significance. In the chapter on Attention Deficit Hyperactivity Disorder, there is a good deal stated about how the motor control pathways are parallel to but somewhat earlier developing than the cognitive control pathways and finally the social-emotional control pathways. The second and third control pathways are components of what is involved in Attention Deficit Hyperactivity Disorder; we therefore used to regard the frequent co-occurrence with motor control problems as a coincidence. However, much research has demonstrated that one can look at the development of motor control as the "canary in the coal mine" that tends to indicate what the timetable or trajectory of development will be for the other more cognitive-behavioral control circuits. Thus, there is tremendous indirect significance to the documentation of DCD. I myself developed a short examination, later given the name of the Physical and Neurological Examination for Subtle Signs (PANESS) which I first felt driven to create in order to acquire norms (the motor equivalents of height and weight charts) because I was evaluating children for the first time and did not have a clinical background of qualitative experience with the development of motor coordination. Inspired by my desire to substitute some kind of quantitative normative table for boys and girls through the school years, I have since taught this clinical examination to many other professionals, not limited to those with medical degrees; the PANESS has become a research tool applied to various diagnostic situations, most prominently for ADHD, but to a lesser extent for Autistic Spectrum Disorder (ASD). In its most recent application, the PANESS is being studied as a "biomarker" for the brain as a baseline for athletes and as a post-concussion recovery indicator.

> Motor development has indirect significance as a "canary in the coal mine" of how myelination for the other rapid controls will follow, permitting "cool" and then "hot" executive function to mature.

6

Executive Function

The term executive function has been spoken of very often in a unitary fashion, but in fact, it is an umbrella term, as is cognitive control, for a group of mental processes, not all of which are so "higher order" in the rather exalted manner in which they are often regarded. It would be preferable to use the plural form, "executive functions" or "cognitive control processes." I also recommend reserving the term "metacognition" not as a synonym for the entire domain of executive functions but rather for the very final step in development of the domain. Inhibition, something that is also a component of the domain of motor control, is a very basic aspect of early development of executive function. Working memory, as can be demonstrated nonverbally in laboratory animal experiments, is the next relatively early basic component of executive functions. In human beings, there is a developmental trajectory in which inhibition "checks in" at a simple level towards the end of the year of life, while working memory also enters the picture very gradually, perhaps not so apparent until there is enough inhibition that it is possible to see at preschool age. Gradually there are milestones marking blossoming of what are commonly called "higher order" mental processes (organization and planning) that exert control over an individual's actions and emotional expressions in a manner we refer to as goal-oriented. The executive functions we subsume under "behavior regulation" include inhibition and shifting, as well as a very special case of inhibition, emotional control over overt expressions such as immediate "emoting" (crying, yelling, aggressive words or actions). The cognitive controls include initiating (getting started), sustaining, and shifting (which can be thought of as a two-step sequence of inhibiting an ongoing activity in order to initiate another one). This is my analogy to the automobile "gear shift"; the processes implied in paying attention, what is referred to often as executive attention (Initiate, Sustain, Inhibit, and Shift). The components that "check in" later are higher order functioning; these are planning (across the time dimension, especially as regards time management), organization (which includes spaces and objects, organization of materials and pieces of work physically embodied), and still later, self-monitoring or checking back over that which has been planned and organized in order to see whether a goal has been met. Very late in the developmental trajectory, possibly as late as college age, there arises true "metacognition" in the executive domain, which means that a person has self-knowledge of his or her cognitive strengths and weaknesses. Metacognition involves a complex ability to plan and organize towards a goal with self-knowledge of strengths and how strategies can be utilized to circumvent or compensate for weaknesses of the person's non-executive cognitive endowments, such as language, visuospatial, or motor abilities.

This entire chapter is devoted to the neuropsychological domain of executive function (EF) and executive dysfunction

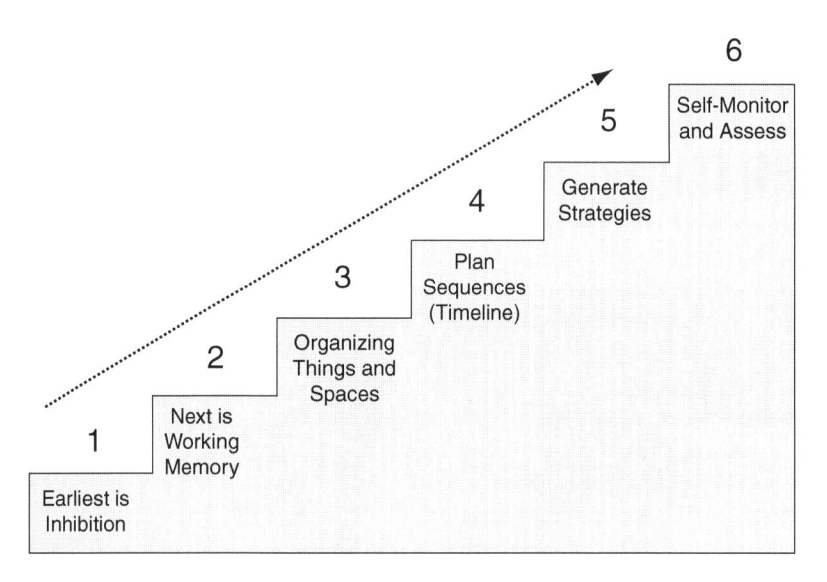

Figure 6.1 Developmental stages of executive functions.

(EDF). I have to explain all the time that there is no diagnosis of "executive function disorder." This is why I prefer to talk about EDF by analogy with using other terms with the prefix "dys" like "dyslexia" and "dyspraxia." Executive function has become such a popularized term that for quite a few years now, clinics such as mine have been consulted by parents asking whether this clinic makes a diagnosis of "executive function disorder." I repeat, there is no such existing diagnosis, but I can explain to educators that EDF is a cognitive control processing problem, a source of underachievement in school.

Widely publicized for the past quarter of a century, the term "executive function" refers not to a diagnosis but control processes that can be summarized as "cognitive control" (currently referred to as "cool executive function") and "social-emotional control" (currently referred to as "hot executive function"). The chapter on motor coordination has already referred to the fact that the motor control circuits in the brain are located in a parallel fashion to the cognitive control and the social-emotional control circuits. (For those who like to hear about brain terminology, these circuits are lined up in such a way that they are loops going both ways between the frontal lobe and both the basal ganglia and the cerebellum.) The motor control is not considered part of "executive function," but is a good model for understanding EF because it is clear that coordination in the motor domain involves "how and when" actions are accomplished. Cognitive control also involves "how and when" more complicated actions are carried out, and the same is certainly true of the emotional control circuits. It is also interesting that there is no sudden appearance of each one of these circuits, each one begins from early in life and follows a trajectory to a final plateau of "good enough for life" that occurs in the following order: first, motor control on average reaches this mature plateau around age 15 (with a normal range of plus/minus three years), cognitive control around age 25 and social-emotional control in the early 30s, probably around age 32. (I'm sorry that it is not completely in intervals of ten years, with "five" as the second digit in each of these ages, as it would be easier to memorize "15–25–35," but the facts are simply not supportive of that simplification.) The fact that the motor control circuitry, located parallel to the two different EF circuits, matures earlier is an important way in which we can probe the developmental predictors and identify those children who are at risk for "immaturity" of EF and would benefit from modified expectations and increased supports or scaffolding.

To illustrate that we do not acquire these EF circuits all at once, the other important "hot" or social-emotional control components of EF have been the focus of work on young prekindergarten children. The famous "marshmallow test" comes to mind, a test in which a child is told that if he or she, seated at a table on which there is a single marshmallow, can wait for an examiner to return to the room, he or she will receive a second marshmallow; but if he or she consumes the marshmallow left on the table in front of the child, there will not be this reward. All kinds of interpersonal situations at a young age require a certain basic level of "hot" executive function (social-emotional control) most prominently inhibition.

Cognitive controls in the service of problem-solving also begin very young. One of the most ingenious demonstrations of the beginning of executive function is an experiment with babies between 6 and 12 months of age, in which a baby is seated on the lap of the mother or caregiver and shown a teddy bear inside a completely transparent Plexiglas box that is open on the side but which looks to the baby like it is directly visible behind the transparent surface that faces the infant. Up to about nine months, the average baby will reach directly forward to try to grab the teddy bear and will, of course, meet with the barrier of the Plexiglas. The remarkable "baby step" of EF is that of inhibition, whereby at around that age of nine months on average, the infant's hand will reach out, stop and begin to explore the entire outer surface of the Plexiglas container, thereby discovering the side that is open and being able to reach in and get the teddy bear. (I suppose one could say that this is planning as well as inhibition, but certainly the inhibitory step seems to be necessary before the exploratory phase we may call planning starts to work.)

Inhibition indeed is the basic platform component of executive function that starts before the first birthday and continues to increase with development, remaining applicable to all aspects of the other control processes contained under the term EF.

It is still not unanimous among experts on the topic of ADHD to say that EDF is associated with ADHD; not that there is often demonstrable EDF in children and adolescents with ADHD but that EDF is not confined to or specific for ADHD, being a feature of ASD and anxiety, among other clinical situations. There are two strategies I have often used when talking to parents to make them understand executive function (synonymous with cognitive control). One is the analogy of the automobile. The person's intellectual or cognitive strengths, his or her various "ingredients" of abilities/talents, are "under the hood of the car"; like the engine and all of the other parts that are usually not very familiar to most of us who drive the car, but to the auto mechanic are what actually provide the potential for the car to go. The controls, the EF domain, are what we use all the time when we are drivers; there are brakes (inhibition), as well as the steering wheel and accelerator, and we all know that there has to be a very good balance between when the brakes are used and the accelerator is required. We also have either gear shifts or some automatic transmission that at least allows us to select whether we are going forward or in reverse. We have lots of other controls that have to do with weather conditions; our windshield wipers for the rain, our defrosting mechanism, our lights, even temperature controls for the comfort of the operator, and so on. So the analogy here would be that the nonexecutive "ingredients" (perceptual, language, memory, all kinds of other specific abilities of the brain), the potentials needed for various kinds of learning, all of these are "under the hood" of the car. The control panel and the mechanisms inside the car that the driver uses, all of these would be the controls or, collectively as the dashboard, the executive functions.

The other analogy one could use would be that of the cook in the kitchen. The intellectual endowments, talents, or cognitive capabilities of the individual in a nonexecutive sense, would be all of the many kinds of food and seasonings (again "ingredients") in the cabinets or in the refrigerator. The recipes that must be followed, including the feature of "looking ahead" at the recipe (for example, to take the butter out of the refrigerator or freezer in a timely fashion if the recipe calls for room temperature butter) are in the EF domain. In this analogy, we have a well-stocked kitchen as the nonexecutive "ingredients," while the recipes and the timing, planning, and procedures are the executive functions (again, synonymous with cognitive controls).

The overview is that executive functions are core skills that are not specific to any one module of ability, not limited to application to any one aspect of cognition, to language, to visual-spatial skills, to interpersonal-social skills, indeed to any of our specific abilities. EF refers to core skills we call "domain-general," critical for all these aspects of our endowment to be developed and contribute to our physical and mental health as well as to our success in school and in life. EF represents a group of dynamic processes that depend on connections among brain regions that will with experience activate together; in addition, these connections and activations shift dynamically in different tasks and different contexts. It makes it very difficult to measure executive function in the developing young person by testing using EF challenges at any given time, especially since the very environments in which we test EF tend to be structured in such a way that the examiner provides instructions, positive reinforcements, and clearly defined limits, such that make all but the most

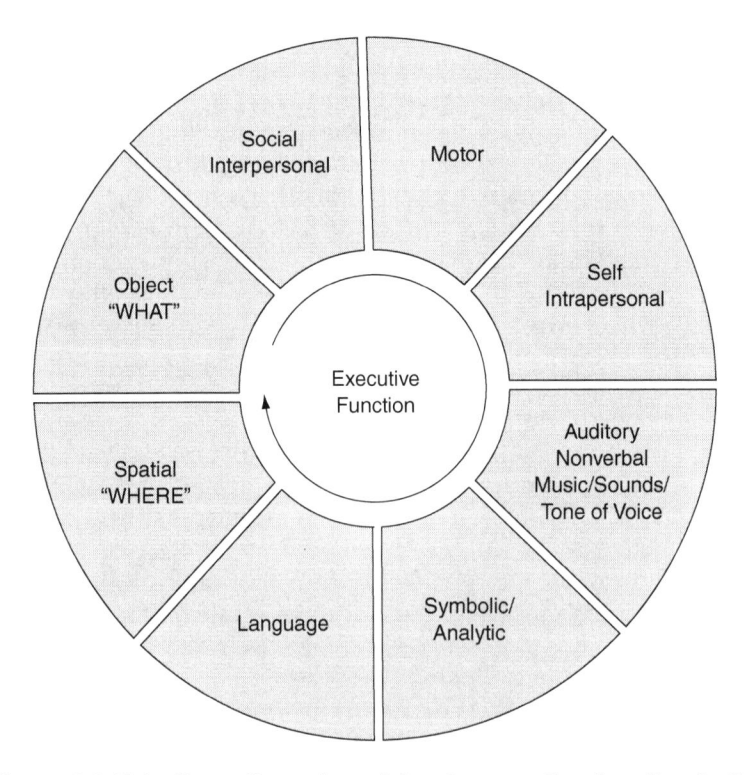

Figure 6.2 This "Lazy Susan" model puts executive function in the middle, the controlling revolving component, with specific abilities in "trays" from which coordinations or compensations may be selected.

severely impaired youngster able to perform within normal limits. In older adolescents and adults, EDF emerges only when they are "on their own," with expectations that they can be fully independent and self-regulatory.

There's also the difficulty inherent in making a distinction what belongs under the EF "umbrella" and what is called the general intelligence factor. It is especially the cool variety of EF that has the most to do with school achievement, and overlaps with what is foundational to IQ. Again, this is most true in the assessment setting, where what has been said about the facilitation of EF performance is equally true of intelligence (IQ) testing. Recent versions of IQ tests have teased out some EF components, so that the professional who reads reports can see that Processing Speed and Working Memory Scales within the IQ scores can reflect EDF (in contrast to the Verbal, Perceptual, and Reasoning Scales). Neuropsychologists strive to add challenges to EF in assessment tools by introducing necessary approaches to novelty, flexible problem-solving, and independent planning/organizational strategies not previously rehearsed.

The basis for the dynamic development of executive function may be found in the fact that the networks of the immature brain tend to be local or connected within short distances; neurons that are neighbors are more fully connected and only gradually become more remotely connected according to a developmental process that takes time and is related both to activation by usage and to the underlying mechanism of myelination (please see chapter on brain development). During the dynamic processes that always include interaction with the environment, the networks of connections become increasingly segregated from each other, but both the integration and the capacity for switching between the networks increase.

Another way to summarize executive function is that it represents the transformation of the human being from a "reflexive" into a "reflective" human being. The example given of inhibition providing the "pause that refreshes" in order to facilitate exploration and goal achievement is one of the compelling images of how a reflex (to reach for the desired teddy bear) must be inhibited before there is a successful exploration, and working memory is needed on a very basic level in order for the infant to keep track of what surface has been explored before discovering the one side that is open and accessible.

It has already been stated that there is no such thing as "executive function disorder," but rather that EDF can exist within and across many different "official" diagnoses. One of the most important things to realize is that anxiety itself can impair executive function. Anxiety can operate through the connection between the emotional brain (for example, the amygdala), which can flood the frontal system with excessive levels of a neurotransmitter that pushes the system into the impaired side of the executive domain, resulting in EDF. Either anxiety alone or anxiety added on top of one of the other neurodevelopmental conditions encapsulated by what we are here considering as "the inconvenient brain" can be a generator of EDF. For example, a child who has a very pure dyslexia profile can develop so much anxiety about school that parents and teachers begin to raise the question of whether that child also has ADHD. While this may be true in about a third of children with dyslexia, there is also the possibility in the other two-thirds that school-performance-based anxiety is causing the executive dysfunction, which includes what appears to be inattentiveness, and may be confused with ADHD, an incorrect diagnosis.

Inhibition is absolutely essential in order for attention to be paid to education. Let's face it, much of education is not particularly engaging or attractive and involves the acquisition of skills that become the automatic infrastructure of more interesting learning; but at every level there is some work that is required that is not intrinsically engaging or attractive to most children. Allocation of attention to educational tasks and chores requires inhibiting the desire to be doing something more attractive. (I have often felt that we are misleading ourselves by using the term "distraction" when we are really talking about "attraction.")

Neurologically, the most basic constituents of executive function are response inhibition, working memory (both verbal and visual-spatial), and response preparation. Processing speed is affected by response preparation. Processing speed is a term that is used by and familiar to educators and psychologists who perform assessments used to communicate an individual's characteristics to educators. So is working memory, although the general understanding of working memory seems to be somewhat confounded with short-term memory or by thinking that working memory is some kind of amalgam of short- and long-term memory. (A simple way to capture the short-term/working distinction is that short-term memory would be represented by repeating digits forward after hearing them, while saying digits backward represents working memory.)

Processing speed is important in the development of fluency in reading and in other academic skills (think of those "mad minutes" of performing arithmetic facts). When there is poor fluency based on slow processing, higher level processes can compete with very basic ones that should be automatic for time-limited resources and create a bottleneck in skills such as reading and arithmetic.

To return to the conceptualization of the important executive component of working memory that is so often impaired in many different kinds of childhood developmental problems, it is good to visualize the basic research because we can learn from research using primates what is recorded directly from certain cells (neurons) that really are "working memory cells" in the brain. Visualize a monkey looking at an array of 180 degrees around him, the array being made of little Christmas lights. The monkey is rewarded for looking at a particularly located Christmas light. Then things get more difficult; the monkey is rewarded for looking at a position where a particular specific Christmas light was on but has been off for a few seconds. During the few seconds between the light being on and the monkey moving his eyes to the spot where the light was a few seconds ago, there are cells we recognize as working memory cells that are firing off and preserving that spatial information in order for it to be responded to by eye movement cells. This spatial working memory can be thought of as the "hyphen" in between what has been seen and the response to what was seen but is no longer present.

Working memory temporarily retains information between an experience that no longer exists and a response that must be made. Working memory may be necessary to guide and control behavior. In a more complex way, items have to be retrieved from long-term memory and held in working memory in order for appropriate actions to take place.

As is the case with processing speed affecting fluency, which in turn affects reading comprehension, so it is also true that working memory affects reading comprehension.

Working memory is also extremely important in performing all kinds of mathematical problem-solving, even that which we see as arithmetic. In a multistep operation, what has just been done has to be "kept in mind" in order to move the sequence of the calculation to the next step. Again, developmental progression occurs dynamically across a remarkable long span of life, the "hot" component reaching into those years beyond 30; there is a very long period of opportunity for the environment to either enhance or damage the development of EF. What we have said about anxiety applies to stress having an adverse effect upon the development of EF, and of course chaotic, unstructured environments fail to provide the inputs to the brain necessary for the construction of these networks. Comparative biology shows us that inhibitory control, in evolutionary terms, is a basic capacity that is conserved across species. This occurs even in relatively solitary animals but becomes more and more a survival mechanism as social group size increases. It had been found that disorganized chaotic households, often resulting from low socioeconomic status, impede the ability to promote the early aspects of executive function such as inhibitory control. There is great opportunity to either enhance EF or derail it to EDF, and the earlier the derailment, the more that brain structure in terms of missed connections can become suboptimal; we cannot look at EF or EDF simply as genetically programmed brain processes that will develop independent of the "epigenetic" influences from the environment.

> Executive function is a domain of brain development that is complex (it involves "cool" and "hot" controls); it unfolds in stages, always relevant to every school problem and every effective intervention; executive dysfunction has many sources aside from ADHD and many impacts.

We also have to examine how our educational expectations might be running ahead of what is developmentally appropriate; this may well be an escalation of school stress that can result in EDF.

I will be bringing up EDF in other chapters as a contributor to specific academic problems and how interventions or accommodations in school may be restorative of EF. To end this chapter, I would like to state that probably recognition and understanding of EF, EDF, and of what may be pseudo-EDF (actually immature EF prematurely expected) may be of greatest importance in protecting some children from being interpreted as "lazy," or "irresponsible," or "unmotivated" in a moralizing frame of reference. To optimize their realization of their potential and to be well-adjusted, these children should be understood as standing in need of adult support in terms of modeling, guiding, and scaffolding "how and when" to accomplish tasks.

7

• • • • •

Autistic Spectrum Disorder (ASD)

The high functioning portion of the autistic spectrum was what my clinic has been concerned with, as the clinic was devoted to core academic problems and was by no means an "Autism Center." Especially when Asperger Syndrome was introduced (see later in this chapter), children with subtle school problems but many precocious academic skills began to appear in my clinic, even if they were being followed for years in "Autism Center" facilities. Recently, Asperger Syndrome is no longer a separate diagnostic category officially used in this country, although nonprofessional patients, families, and even some schools continue to find it a useful term somewhat separate from high functioning Autistic Spectrum Disorder (ASD). Health care professionals have to concede that they are no longer allowed to write as a diagnosis Asperger Syndrome, now that there is no recognition of its distinctive course, "drummed out of the corps." (As of DSM-5, this was decided; the Committee on ASD cited studies reporting that there wasn't a difference between high functioning autism and Asperger significant enough to warrant there being a separate diagnosis; this was based on data on children 8–12 years old and dismissed the course in preschool years.) Publications concerning the history of Dr. Asperger, who apparently was a Nazi or at least a Nazi collaborator, have further dampened enthusiasm for the use of the term; yet, having been among the first in this country to meet Dr. Lorna Wing when she introduced the work of Dr. Asperger in English, and having seen children whose excellent language development delayed recognition of their core autistic qualities, I am not entirely convinced that the syndrome should be discarded. Perhaps a new name, free of the eponym "Asperger," should be considered.

From an educational point of view, the Asperger group tends to learn and remember certain kinds of information, much of it very useful for academic achievement, better than any other group included under the title, "Inconvenient Brains." Learning and memory strengths in the high end of ASD will introduce the subject of different *kinds* of learning and memory. There's a kind of learning and memory that's called *declarative* and is much of what we use in education and our store of information about our own lives. Pieces of information, facts, accumulated from my daily life, like my date of birth and Social Security number, are referred to as declarative memories but are not as rich as the *episodic* memory, our multisensory "video" autobiography. Learning facts in school is dependent upon declarative memory, but we also learn procedures, skills, and actions, e.g., how to tie shoelaces, how to type, how to play the piano, how to move our mouths in response to certain letters of the alphabet. (Yes, learning to read, especially using phonics, is acquired and retained in *procedural* learning and memory. It is a skill and can be acquired in a foreign language you don't understand or speak as long as the alphabetic principle is used to "decode.") Children with Asperger or high functioning ASD have excellent declarative and some kinds of procedural learning strengths (reading, playing musical instrument, drawing, but not usually athletics). It is not clear whether their episodic or autobiographical learning and memory are strengths, which is intriguing because there may be an intersection between these and social cognition; much research remains to be done on this topic.

So, basically, what is the autistic spectrum, which began its history as Early Infantile Autism? Well, at Johns Hopkins, visible from my office at Kennedy Krieger Institute, Dr. Leo Kanner studied a group of 11 children for whom he introduced this label, "Early Infantile Autism." At about the same time, an Austrian, Dr. Asperger, towards the end of World War II, so he wasn't certainly getting read very much, described the syndrome that bears his name. It wasn't until 1981 that Dr. Lorna Wing wrote about Dr. Asperger's publication now translated into English; what he described was essentially a different developmental trajectory leading to in mid-childhood a clinical picture similar to high functioning autism. What is important is the normal or precocious language acquisition, the distinctive feature of Asperger Syndrome. This is one reason why I disagree with Asperger Syndrome having been discarded in the DSM-5. I cannot believe that, even if children by the age of eight share social impairment and a restricted repertoire of repetitive behavior, if some can talk at two and some can't talk until six years of age (after intensive applied behavior analysis/language-centered therapy), four years later, that really doesn't imply an important neurodevelopmental difference. No matter that the MRIs don't look different at ages above eight years or that neuropsychological tests reveal no significant differences, the pathway or trajectory, and probably the developmental mechanism, was different. The lack of research data on younger children is due to the fact that children with atypical brains are too young to be studied by any of our research techniques because they're unable to cooperate with MRIs or formal neuropsychology. Then we collect data after the period when the groups of children probably show (but we can't see) differences and base conclusions on mid-childhood, when they're already looking much more similar to each other.

Turning to the clinical experience: ASD diagnoses that are reasons for atypical children to be referred to Autism Centers are not for academic issues but for age-inappropriate or odd social behaviors. Most of the time, the behaviors prompting referrals were odd, disquieting, or "inappropriate" not in a combative or aggressive way but more withdrawn nonparticipation or eccentric preoccupation. Such children might be observed in potentially social or play time spending recess walking around the playground repetitively, alone, unaware of looking "weird" either doing nothing, or muttering phrases to themselves, or lining up sticks along the perimeter of the fence. In class, this child might be doing math or some other subject selectively, or might be in all academic subjects achieving well. Their school behavior may be "weird" but not necessarily disruptive unless there occurs something out of the ordinary, a deviation from routine, or something that according to their rigid expectations goes wrong. However, I will allude later to the fact those who are referred for possible Asperger Syndrome often do not turn out to fit that diagnosis, despite superficial resemblance to some of the behaviors; a careful developmental history points in another direction, to another type of "inconvenient brain."

What are the core deficits of any person in the autistic spectrum (ASD)? Atypical communication and social interaction, and a restricted repetitive repertoire of behavior. (The last of these, the restrictive repetitive repertoire, was contributed in that form by me and, I am proud to say, has survived intact through several revisions of the DSM.) The more intelligent the child is the more that their stereotyped, repetitive, restricted repertoire can be that they talk on a topic incessantly. (This is the verbal equivalent of the commonly depicted repetitions of those with low functioning ASD, such as flapping their arms, jumping up and down, banging their heads, grunting or vocalizing). Those in the ASD with strong language skills may talk on a certain subject like a "broken record." They seem to be "captured" (obsessed) by some very narrow subject; for example, preoccupation with learning the schedules of all the airlines that fly out of a local airport or the exact positions of the heavenly constellations each day. The restricted repetitive repertoire component is distinctive but can be seen as an extreme form of what is typical. (You know how a lot of five- and six-year-old boys get obsessed with dinosaurs?) But, it's a question of degree and duration, although after years the obsession may shift. It's a question of how hard it would be to get those with ASD to shift flexibly off of this topic, how readily you can entice them elsewhere. There are also children of normal intelligence who exhibit stereotypies when over-aroused but are not in the autistic spectrum; many of these have Attention Deficit Hyperactivity Disorder and can actually stop stereotypies when medicated with stimulants.

All children in the autistic spectrum demonstrate impairment of reciprocal social interaction; their communication deficiency is not necessarily in words understood or expressed but involves atypical nonverbal communication. They may use either no rise and fall of vocal tone (*prosody* is the formal term) at all, very flat voices, or they might use exaggerated "babyish" loud vocal intonation, which means they sound like much younger children. Typically, vocal modulation grows more subtle, just as handwriting grows smaller. (We go from kindergarten wide ruled paper to college ruled.) In our culture, it is expected that as you learn from your social setting, you're supposed to control your voice within a narrow amplitude and adjust its volume to settings. There are cultural and age-related differences in this modulation. What makes those with ASD sound "weird" is not just what words they're saying but how their voices carry the words in a social-emotional communicative context.

In both school and social life, those "in the Spectrum" fail at one of the only clear examples of true parallel processing "multi-tasking" (tasks that you habitually do at the same time), when you process both the words I'm saying and my tone of voice, integrating these two separate streams of auditory perceptions. Those in the ASD category are terrible at that. It may be just because they're specifically terrible at processing the vocal tone, but you really have to say in so many words explicitly what you are feeling. If it's a dual simultaneous words-and-feelings message, they're not "getting it."

ASD involves qualitative impairments in communication: 1) delay in development of spoken language; 2) marked impairment in the ability to initiate and sustain conversation; and 3) stereotyped and repetitive use of language or a language that is idiosyncratic, meaning that they use words according to self-determined meanings. I love this example from Dr. Asperger's original paper translated by Lorna Wing; a boy thought that the word he was asked to define, "independent," meant "to jump into the deep end of the pool," in-de-pen-dent. (We do have nonliteral words like "understanding"—standing under what? What do you mean we're "understanding?") Children with ASD tend to listen to words very concretely as vocabulary develops and give them their own meaning, often literal. Again, this is because they're not really paying attention to how other people are using the word. They're not picking up their vocabulary in the context of social interaction. And then, of course, they never pick up the kinds of things that "tweens" and, obviously, teens pick up from the peer group, which is all the generation-specific "lingo." (For example, I just found out that LOL has gone out of style and now people write "haha" on texts. I mean, it's changing so fast, and all of a sudden LOL is "out.") You can really see how "tweens" and teens who are "in the Spectrum" are not going to be fluent in their social lives, whereas a youngster with ADHD may be "with it" in the linguistic shifts but then use words inappropriately, at the wrong time or with the wrong person. The other aspect of communication impaired in ASD is the nonverbal communicative "envelope" of vocal intonation, facial expression and "body language." This is the impaired and severely delayed communication shared even by the verbal (Asperger).

Then there is lack of social-emotional reciprocity; often those with ASD express their needs but they don't exhibit awareness that the other person also has needs. For example, sometimes they will pinch (although, of course, all children sometimes pinch or bite or do something to other children), but will have no idea that the pinched person will feel the same way that they would feel a pinch. There's something missing from their processing the expressed emotions of others. And that goes under this unnecessarily academic name (excuse my editorializing) of "Theory of Mind." (Why is it a theory? Why "mind" and not "feeling"?) It's such a basic human feeling, empathy. Empathy is somehow just knowing you're a person/I'm a person! "Theory of Mind" makes it sound like something very advanced or metacognitive, meaning "knowing about knowledge," which seems to me too conscious, too developmentally beyond the stage when shared humanity comes alive in human beings. Typical toddlers who are still on a very prerational, preverbal level and wouldn't have any sense of what we call morality will still show that basic empathy. The way researchers test for "Theory of Mind" is through perception of a series of unemotional scenes and *verbal* responses to *verbal* questions about who knew what happened. And some excellent researchers have shown that loss of "Theory of Mind" can occur after traumatic injury to the brain's frontal lobes, so it's not specific to autism/ASD. People in the autistic spectrum do display empathy for very dramatic or explicitly described distress of others, but at lower arousal day-to-day levels of experience empathy is not evident in their behavior.

As you would predict, difficulty with teasing causes disruptive reactions in those with ASD. (Of course, nowadays I have trouble delineating "teasing" because everything negative of any degree is called "bullying.") Currently, those in the Spectrum are disadvantaged when there is little taught in the way of manners; it's getting difficult to remain "politically correct" when we all are treading on eggshells as to what we are allowed to say or supposed to say. Some of the ASD-related social and communication skills can be temporarily masked by advanced verbal skills, especially when in elementary school, in rule-governed settings interacting with adults; adults may be very much impressed with how knowledgeable or even polite (if well-taught in old-fashioned phrases) they are. When visiting a science museum, a child "in the Spectrum" (Asperger) may, if alone with the parent, look impressive, even precocious. Even as small an added social "load" as taking a friend along to the science museum may reveal failure on the simplest action, like not realizing when you're blocking your friend's view of the exhibit, an adjustment just to let the other person see what's going on, much less turn and share the experience with advanced verbal "joint attention."

How do you make a diagnosis of ASD? The dominant methods are the Autism Diagnostic Interview (ADI) and the Autism Diagnostic Observation System (ADOS): one of them is an interview (ADI) and the other one is an observation of the child (ADOS). Again, documenting qualitative impairment and atypical social interactions is very important, encompassing nonverbal behaviors, not just language. Even if within the family there is some typical interaction, if one probes deeply, there will be failure to develop other relationships.

Quite often, children with ASD do have relationships with their parents; they may be very infantile relationships. They may not be seeking more independence as typical children do, gradually pushing away from their parents; they may remain too dependent and then retain an inappropriately "sticky" parent–child bond. It's difficult to tease out just how much the parent is perpetuating the immature and clinging behavior, with its excessive demands for attention, by overresponding to the child expressing the need for this more infantile relationship. The main theme is that those with ASD are nonexploratory. It's almost as though words like "failure to shift," "inflexible," or "resistant to change" represent withdrawal from the typical fundamental drive to explore and become independent seen in typical human children, even in practically every other kind of atypical "disabled" child. The distinctive exception with ASD is this aversion to exploration, which can look like anxiety. I have a theory that you can put a preschooler with ASD in a playroom and watch him or her grab hold of one toy and keep doing the same thing with the toy over and over again, whereas a typical preschooler is going to be playing a reasonable amount of time with one toy, perhaps explore another toy, or then try out different ways of playing with that toy. (Those with ADHD would be like butterflies, not staying long with any one toy, but "flitting" from toy to toy.) You can observe two young children, one with ASD and one with ADHD, both of whom could be described as "hyperactive." If you just put an actimeter (measuring movement) on them, the difference would emerge when you looked at the activity paths. The path of the one with ADHD would be all over the place, randomly hyperexploratory; with ADHD, they're in "Brownian" motion, like little molecules are bouncing around. In contrast, the one with ASD is repeatedly active on a single track, practically wearing a trodden path in the carpet.

A lack of spontaneous seeking to share experiences is one of the earliest signs documented in research on ASD. Unlike typical infants, those with ASD do not show what's called "joint attention." If they're playing with a toy and Mommy's sitting next to them, they don't point or turn and use eye contact to try to get the mother to look at the toy with them. They don't try to engage the mother's involvement in their experiences, even if joyful and smiling. This lack of instinctive sharing by recruiting others to "joint attention," is one of the earliest and best replicated ASD characteristics.

In developmental diagnosis, those whom we used to call "Asperger Syndrome" seem great with language so to place them "in the Spectrum" what do you see in social interaction or social communication? For example, in retrospect, when you can look at old videos, you see babies who, even as young as six months on their mother's lap will sit facing outward and use the mother as a chair; but unlike others of that age won't squirm around and try to engage with the mother. Typical six-month-old infants pull on the mother's hair, glasses, earring, often smiling playfully in an exploratory and affectionate interpersonal way. The "future" ASD babies just sit facing forward and reach for an object in front, outwardly, just using the comfortable chair-like enveloping lap and arms of the mother, without engaging joint attention or other interaction with the mother. This is strikingly atypical, even in some of those who are very intelligent and develop speech, language, and even precocious reading very easily.

At all levels of cognitive ability, all "in the Spectrum" really want things around them to be the same; they get agitated or hysterical if a parent drives to school a different way (because there's construction work and she has to take a detour). They respond frantically to furniture rearrangements or minor schedule changes. They are rigid about schedules and expect the order and duration of activities to stay the same, so even having to go to a dental appointment after school will cause a "meltdown," just because it is not a routine daily occurrence.

With ASD, especially those I still refer to as fitting Asperger, there are three- and four-year-olds you see who love to play house, commanding "you be this and you be that and I'll be that." Now when I recall some Asperger-diagnosed five-year-old referrals, one whom I remember well showed atypical play based on his having memorized every single word of *Beauty and the Beast*, the Disney movie. On play dates with him, children who acted out the general gist were not well received; he insisted they had to say the exact correct lines. He would insist on going back to the script's beginning, upset by the paraphrasing of his playmate. "No, no, no, you didn't say the right thing; we have to start over and say it right!" Needless to say, this was not enjoyable to others and resulted in early ending of the play date. This "tape recorded" level of "play" illustrates lack of understanding on two levels: 1) even if they had watched it 25 times, the other child might not have it memorized; and 2) the other child may not want to play this way, may not find verbatim reenactment enjoyable.

Returning to the role of play, we see it's difficult to teach children "in the Spectrum" to play games that involve the element of chance like rolling dice. They'll learn to play chess but they won't learn to play Monopoly, because with chess there are these defined rules; but with Monopoly you have to roll the dice and you might be a "loser" by chance. Despite some interest in others, this involves assigning others to be meeting needs (parents), enacting specific roles (peers), or being an audience to monologues. Other persons play a role, but it's not a reciprocal role. When others are not interested in what they have to say (often a long recitation or monologue) they're not monitoring the listeners' body language or facial expression. Lack of understanding occurs when the context is not right for the topic of obsessive interest. Very concrete understanding of language hampers them; if a school has what they call a "Spirit Club," those in the Spectrum will think that has something to do with religion rather than school spirit, another example of missing alternative meanings of words that are context dependent.

Persistent preoccupation with parts or features of objects can characterize anyone "in the Spectrum." The one I can never forget is an adult man whom I saw (when I was at the National Institutes of Health [NIH] and was in a collaboration with an adults-with-ASD research project), an adult man with Asperger Syndrome, who was totally preoccupied with fabrics, particularly whether or not it was cotton. He got into trouble because if he got in the elevator, he would lean over and start fingering others' clothing, asking earnestly, "Is this 100 percent cotton?" You can imagine that a young adult male starting to pick up and feel the hem of a woman's skirt for its fabric was going to get him into trouble!

In the "sensory" domain, those in the autistic spectrum will often communicate distress or act aversive to certain sensory stimuli or overly attracted to others. This is an odd set of reactions.

Many of those with ASD can't stand loud noises that occur abruptly in the environment, but love the kinds of mechanical noises that you and I would consider to be boring, like a fan, refrigerator, or some appliance electrically plugged in that makes a background hum. Loud, sudden, unanticipated noises set off something like a panic reaction, while low volume repetitive noise is pleasing. Sameness and predictability are preferred in sensory experience.

A note of caution about what is often assumed to be understood about ASD. The restricted repertoire of the low functioning child with ASD is often called "stimming" (self-stimulating), which is interpreting excessively. We should just describe what we see. They're flapping their hands, jumping up and down, or whatever they're doing repeatedly; we don't know *why* they seem to derive comfort or contentment performing these repetitive behaviors. We should refrain from extrapolating beyond the evidence and admit what remains mysterious.

How common is "the Spectrum?" Recently it has been said that 1 in 68 children are "in the Spectrum." I'm still really very skeptical about the increasing prevalence. I think some of the increase is real (perhaps due to the connection with older fathers), but I think some of it is overenthusiastic diagnosis, because what has happened to our special education services in so many places is that the only really dedicated resources are reserved for "the Spectrum." This is due to very successful lobbying efforts by the parents (and I don't begrudge their children the services), but it's been a sort of "zero sum game" neglecting some of the other disabilities. In particular, it's hard to find a class for the language-impaired, even those with severe language disorders who really need to have substantially separate classes, which they don't get in most public school systems; even private special schools originally founded for the language-impaired are now overwhelmed by demand for the nonverbal child with an ASD diagnosis, sometimes a well-intentioned but deliberately "stretched" diagnosis.

We all know that ASD is the result of anomalous brain development, a neurological disorder. To arrive at this involved a hard-won fight, because although Dr. Kanner believed it was in part something intrinsic, he also made the unfortunate error of saying that often the parents were highly intelligent, highly educated, and rather distant "cool" parents. (I think there may have been a referral bias about who was bringing their children to Dr. Kanner at Johns Hopkins during the later years of the Depression and during World War II.) That was emphasized, unfortunately, by influential psychiatrists, so that there was a long period of viewing autism as caused by cold parents who didn't meet the infant's emotional needs. It was very unfortunate because it blamed so-called "refrigerator" parents, so then therapy spent years trying to get these children to either physically "express their anger" or in the verbal cases participate in psychoanalysis. (When I was in medical school, there were high functioning verbal autistic children undergoing Freudian psychoanalytic treatment at a Harvard Medical School-affiliated psychiatric hospital.)

By the time I became involved with the NIH program on autism in 1981, it really had become evident that the cause was neurological. One of the biggest contributors to that evolution was finding that 25 percent of cases by the time they reached 21 years of age had seizures. This was a big clue; something's going on in the brain if 25 percent of those "in the Spectrum" have seizures, a risk associated with ASD much higher than that of the general population in that age group and higher than with ADHD or Learning Disabilities (LD) developmental "disorders."

By 1980, researchers started doing new imaging (structural/anatomic MRI) with results best summarized as inconsistent or in conflict. Nonconcordance raises the issue of selection of those included in the research, both in terms of age and level of function. (I have always taught my trainees to start reading a research report by searching in the Methods section to pin down exactly "about whom we are speaking.") Just as there was probably a referral bias for Dr. Leo Kanner, there could be a recruitment bias for research using any technique; informed consent is the second "filter" after recruitment, so each study is limited to those whose parents agree to participate/have their child participate. Then there is the problem of capacity of the child to lie still in the MRI scanner, eliminating younger or lower functioning children. Even more of a complication is that imaging studies may show a finding at one age and then when scanning the same children at an older age, will no longer show the same finding but a new and different fining. Anomalous brain development may take you off course in a different, unexpected way and longitudinal studies are difficult to perform, much less obtain funding to carry out over many years.

There are no clinical tests, not even MRIs that classify as ASD individual cases, even though research MRIs show ASD group differences from typical scans. In other words, you can't refer an individual child for an MRI or a blood test or an EEG that will confirm or even suggest the diagnosis of ASD. There are certain conditions, genetic or infectious disease, that are more likely to show a picture of ASD but account for a small percent of diagnoses.[1] The underlying causes are entirely separate issues from the clinical pictures which professionals and families must confront. Early social and language development is the best predictor of outcome; being able to talk by age six is a very important prognostic sign. If you remain nonverbal at six, you're in the worst prognostic group. Even with optimal treatment (language therapy, behavior modification) there tends to be a flattening off or plateau of improvement by the time the challenges of puberty set in; but this, again, may be only partially "hormonal" while largely to do with how much increased demand there is for the very behaviors that autistic individuals are not endowed with: flexibility, the greater complexity of being social in that age group, and greater independence of action. Supervisors and rules still exist, but "cover" less of life as one reaches adolescence.

I must detour from my usual clinical emphasis to affirm that immunizations do not cause ASD. It's unbelievable, after all the time and money spent on research studies addressing this concern, that so many young or new parents "believe" in this discredited connection; one of the most shameful episodes in medical publishing was that such a claim, autism caused by immunizations, was ever published in a major journal and amplified by mass media. Even after retraction of the report by the prestigious journal, exposing the original report's flaws, devoting resources to investigating the possibilities, the myth persists. The consequences go far beyond ASD, to all children, when we have seen outbreaks of measles make a reappearance in the USA. Even well-educated people have become distrustful of vaccinations, which poses a health risk to the children of the world.

DSM-5 is "allowing" dual diagnosis, ASD and ADHD. There used to be an exclusion clause such that once you said that a child was "in the Spectrum" they weren't "allowed" to have the diagnosis of ADHD. (The brain didn't "read the book," so whatever is atypical about the brain unfortunately can be anomalous in more than one network; we know that there's a 30 percent overlap between ADHD and learning disability, whichever you start with.) Why did they think that ASD and ADHD couldn't co-occur? I guess it's because ASD is considered the most severe of the developmental diagnoses. Even the minority "in the Spectrum" who are high functioning, without Intellectual Disability, are considered to be much more lifetime severely impaired; they very rarely go out into the general world independent and unprotected. DSM-5 acknowledges that you can identify some "in the Spectrum" who do have ADHD-like behaviors that are complicating the ASD behaviors but can be treated for the ADHD component. My concern is that some children whose ADHD is not recognized early or is poorly treated, who are not welcome in social situations (even preschool play) develop *social learning deprivation* such that they are mistakenly later labeled "in the Spectrum," usually (until recently) thought to have Asperger Syndrome.

What does the future hold for those "in the Spectrum?" You don't see a whole lot of people with ADHD being put on Social Security disability or needing adult services, but with ASD 90 percent of them as adults remain disabled, and a great deal of the cost to society for their care is incurred beyond age 21. Of course, we'd love to achieve early diagnosis and comprehensive intervention to significantly reduce lifetime cost and improve quality of life. Of course, early intervention can include false positives, but we are willing to risk some false positives, because we don't think it harms young children to be given language and behavior modification services. It's a different challenge when you get to those a little older and you include otherwise disabled (language-impaired, nonautistic) children in a class for ASD. Then you really wonder whether you're doing more harm than good. We really shouldn't have to go much beyond the age of two years to make a diagnosis or declare highly suspicious/at risk for "the Spectrum." As opposed to ADHD, which you would find difficult to use as a label before age 3.5 or 4, the "spectrum" risk is atypical rather than immature behavior. You cannot say about ASD as you can for a four-year-old with ADHD, "had this child been younger, the behavior would have seemed normal."

Teaching the child with ASD: for inclusion, what are the strengths? First, these are the verbal and high functioning ones "in the Spectrum." They're very good at rote memorizing and good at retaining concrete literal information. They are detail-oriented almost to a fault. They follow rules, but inflexibly. They thrive on routine and repetition others find boring. (In a way, the computer has shut many of them out of the employment field. We used to have a lot more employment for people who had prodigious memories and tremendous attention to detail, but such jobs are exactly what computers are good at. Actually, employment opportunities have gotten worse for them in the past 30 years.) The challenges for educators dealing with these children are their poor shifting of attention, their overfocus, their inflexibility when problem-solving. You can imagine in a regular classroom this is why so often there is an aide for the child included in order to just move with the program, especially when there are transitions. Additionally, those with ASD, whether or not they have a language disorder, as with the verbal Asperger, may not cope with the speed at which the auditory information flows past; any nonliteral use of language, any tone of voice connoting a message like humor, sarcasm, or displeasure may be lost. It's good teaching to get everything written down for these children and organize it visually to overcome their tendency to overfocus on a single part or feature of a topic. My favorite example of this is the boy who took a test on Egypt (a unit in social studies in middle school) on which he was to write an essay about an important influence in Egyptian culture. The teacher was aiming at a discussion of Egypt's focus on the afterlife, but the boy with Asperger Syndrome just wrote about how the color purple was the sign of high rank, where you got the purple dye from, and who was allowed to wear purple! Somehow that detail, "purple" struck that boy as important and overshadowed larger themes like life after death.

Generalizing is another educational skill those within the autistic spectrum don't exhibit. While they may do well in arithmetic and use facts and procedures memorized, when they have to apply arithmetic to a word problem or apply the hypothesis-testing needed in long division, they may not generalize to varied applications of the same principle or shift flexibly. They may also "melt down" when their own products don't meet their rigid standards, being unable to accept "good enough" because that implies knowing the teacher's expectations rather than an absolute goal.

In summary, much is not understood about what is anomalous about the brains of those identified as belonging to the autistic spectrum. Perhaps more fundamentally, much is not understood about the relevant aspects of cognition, the flexible, adaptive, and social-emotional aspects, and their underlying brain networks. In the immediate future, I am concerned as a clinician about the "elastic" borders of the autistic spectrum, erroneously encompassing children with language impairments or neglected ADHD; over-inclusion is not good for the erroneously encompassed, overburdens the resources needed for the truly included ASD, and threatens to make research less meaningful.

* * * * *

Note

1 Tuberous sclerosis and Fragile X are among established genetic causes of ASD, while over a hundred genes or combinations have been implicated. Maternal infections like "German measles" (rubella) are implicated.

8

Attention Deficit Hyperactivity Disorder (ADHD)

About half of the children and adolescents referred to my clinic come with the question of whether or not they have Attention Deficit Hyperactivity Disorder (ADHD), either as a primary question or as a confirmation (second opinion) request. The term ADHD has existed only since 1980, but I have been seeing similar children going back into the much earlier days of my practice that started in 1970; then the prevailing question was whether the child or adolescent could be diagnosed with what was then called "Minimal Brain Dysfunction."

Many people when asking me about ADHD ask me, "Where are all these children coming from, where did they used to be?" or else, from the standpoint of medications, ask whether there aren't too many prescriptions being written for stimulant medications of various types, since there has been such a proliferation of various forms of the stimulants (old wine in new bottles). The two stimulant classes of proven efficacy are still the same, the amphetamine salts and methylphenidate, the former currently best known as Adderall and the latter known for quite a few years as Ritalin. The point is that there are new names for the diagnoses and drugs and an extension of the age group and types of problems, in terms of symptoms and signs, for which the drugs are prescribed; but even going back into the 1970s, the same types of children were being seen when the question was whether they had "Minimal Brain Dysfunction." Children we now refer to with "ADHD" are very heterogeneous; but equally heterogeneous have been those with the other names applied to the syndrome.

There has been in the history of the syndrome a predominant emphasis on behavioral features, progressing from books about

"Fidgety Phil" or "Disheveled Peter" in European nineteenth-century books, using such quaint terms as "morbid defects of moral control," "post-encephalitic incorrigibility," "Minimum Brain Damage Syndrome," "Hyperkinetic Impulse Disorder," "Hyperactive Child Syndrome," and, in the beginning of my 48 years of clinical work, "Minimal Brain Dysfunction." It is fortunate for me that when I entered the field in 1970, "Minimal Brain Dysfunction" was the umbrella term, because it was the word "brain" in the middle that brought neurologists into the picture, especially where I started my clinical work with children, which was in the state of New Jersey; New Jersey had classes designated for the "neurologically impaired," which meant children who had at least normal intelligence (clearly were not intellectually deficient), but showed a syndrome of hyperactivity, impulsivity, and inattentiveness that we now recognize under the name of ADHD and its various subtypes.

Back in 1962, the National Institute of Neurological Diseases and Stroke (NINDS) defined Minimal Brain Dysfunction as encompassing a range of behavioral and learning problems thought to be associated with central nervous system dysfunctions; hence, the term "brain dysfunction" (the "minimal" is debatable in many cases), which could be manifested by combinations of impairment in perception, motor function, language, memory, attentional control, and impulsivity. To be included there had to be at least average IQ, but the diagnosis clearly encompassed mixed and matched behavioral and cognitive functions. The diagnosis started to be divided up in 1968 when the U.S. Office of Education discussed the categorization in the preparatory phase of what became Public Law 94–142 for special education. Language, memory, and some aspects of perception and motor dysfunction were separated from the "Minimal Brain Dysfunction" components later to be identified as Attention Deficit Hyperactivity Disorder (control of attention and control over impulses). In 1968, a Specific Learning Disability was defined as a disorder in one of several "basic psychological processes" involved in each designated academic area. The Minimal Brain Dysfunction relationship was turned on its head, so that Minimal Brain Dysfunction, although still an umbrella term, most prominently survived in the description of ADHD. This came about because advertisements featured Minimal Brain Dysfunction as the indication for treatment with stimulant medications; hence the over-identification with ADHD. In theory, one still could refer within Minimal Brain Dysfunction to any one of the specific academic learning disabilities (reading, mathematics, writing) but this usage has faded and is rarely revived. The Specific Learning Disability definition still harkened back to the assumptions about Minimal Brain Dysfunction and stated that a learning disability could be traced back to the perceptual handicaps, brain injuries, and developmental "aphasias" (language impairments), but would exclude sensory (vision, hearing), or severe motor handicaps like cerebral palsy and clearly not what was then called "mental retardation" (now called Intellectual Disability) or emotional disturbance. The additional requirement was that appropriate access to schooling and appropriate environmental and socioeconomic advantages had to be present in order for the spotlight to be upon the Specific Learning Disability. But again, Specific Learning Disability implicated brain functions, although referred to as due to "psychological processes." There was a gradual drift away from inclusion of the symptoms of what we now call ADHD from the cognitive or "psychological processing" disorder; in 1980, the American Psychiatric Association's Psychiatric DSM-II confirmed the separation distinguishing Academic Skill Disorders from Attention Deficit Disorders (which then could be ADD or AD[H]D plus or minus hyperactivity). At that time it seemed to go unnoticed that placing "Attention" as the first term in the syndrome was in itself a recognition of its prominent cognitive component. "Minimal Brain Dysfunction" all but disappeared from mention, although in medical settings the term is still occasionally used.

The formative influence of the Minimal Brain Dysfunction era, however, was such as to bring neurologists into the picture, no longer allowing either the psychiatrists or the educators to have exclusive influence over attempts to do research and even to understand clinically the patients who presented with the symptoms of hyperactivity, impulsivity, and/or inattention symptoms. Because of the inclusiveness of the Minimal Brain Dysfunction "umbrella" and because of the State of New Jersey designation of classes for the "neurologically impaired," the neurologist was able to document Minimal Brain Dysfunction in the way most comfortable for a neurologist, the developmental motor examination of the child. If a child is disruptive or underachieving, is there anything about his brain that you can see reflected in his examination that indicates that the brain is not developmentally appropriate for the chronological and intellectual status? The developmental motor examination became a very important "lifeline" for the neurologist to establish "brain factors operating here." Observations that point to certain parts of the brain, not necessarily causations, use motor immaturity to dispute an environmental or emotional factor as the sole cause (although not necessarily eliminated as added cause) of ADHD. The neurologist's knowledge of co-localization of motor control pathways parallel with those of cognitive and emotional control as neighbors led to a significant implication about brain development, even without pointing to any underlying causation. (You couldn't use the motor signs to say *why* the child had some sort of brain problem, but you could say at least that it was not entirely environmental or emotional.)

The growth of research on the neurological basis for what was "hyperactivity" and we now call ADHD was largely attributable to the era of "Minimal Brain Dysfunction," the presence of classes for the neurologically impaired, and the proven utility of the motor examination in a developmental context to implicate "brain factors." Motor control emerged as a very important way of deciding which anatomical and functional magnetic resonance research studies would be most likely to pinpoint regions of interest based on the motor data.

About half of children with ADHD (prepubertal children, that is) will qualify for a diagnosis of Developmental Coordination Disorder. This is not synonymous with saying that the other 50 percent show all of their neurodevelopmental motor capabilities completely up to age expectation. It has been demonstrated for many years that within a school population, children with no problems at all can still have up to four neurodevelopmental anomalies or immaturities. This would include some overflow movements like jaw moving with tongue, some difference of muscle tone between the hands, a winking deficit (meaning the inability to close each eye alone), or some immaturity of balance or gait. More than four "subtle signs," however, are seen in a school survey only among children who show academic problems.

So even if it seems like the diagnosis of ADHD and the use of medications in the student category are "new," in fact they go back a long way, the diagnosis going back into the nineteenth century under a variety of names, and giving stimulant medications to children is also quite old by now, children being medicated since 1937 with mixed amphetamine salts and medicated with

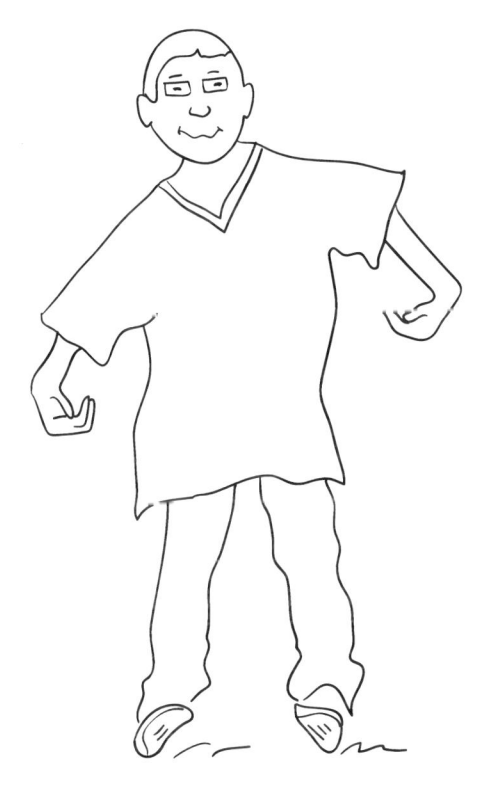

Figure 8.1 Walking on the outsides of the feet, this child shows the unconscious feet-to-hands overflow revealing inhibitory immaturity. This should disappear after nine years of age.

methylphenidate derivatives best known as "Ritalin" since 1948. These are among the best researched and best understood medications given to any age group, and certainly more is known about stimulants given to children than about almost any other group of medications given to children. In any event, neither the prescription of these medications symptomatically nor the fundamental symptom cluster are new, by whatever name; ADHD is only the most recent name.

Fundamentally, under any name, ADHD includes problems of cognitive control and emotional control (or social-emotional control). The psychiatrist is most likely to be consulted for the latter group because disordered social-emotional control is likely to lead to behaviors seen as "disruptive" or "externalizing" ("bad") behavior, as perceived by parents and teachers as indicated by the professional use of terms "disruptive" or "externalizing." However, in 1980 a major change to the new term Attention Deficit Disorder was based upon the work of psychologists who took "hyperactive" children into university laboratories and demonstrated their difficulties with tasks involving sustained attention, introducing a new emphasis on cognitive control. "Attention" as tested or observed put cognitive (specifically attentional) behaviors, long the focus of educators and psychologists closely affiliated with educators, together in a syndrome, equal with psychiatrists' behavioral concerns, social-emotional control deficits. The clinic of a neurologist like me is where the two aspects, cognitive (attentional) and social-emotional (hyperactive/impulsive) are both considered side by side in parallel in the context of the brain. This is why motor control, the traditional focus of the neurologist, connects with the developmental brain map in the neighborhoods of the ADHD controls, cognitive and social-emotional. To fully use this knowledge in clinic, you should see these children when they are prepubertal, because research on the trajectory of motor development shows that most of the time they reach a "good enough for life" plateau of motor controls on average by 15 years of age (plus or minus two years); so that before 13 years of age is the best span during which clinicians can use neurodevelopmental motor control as an index sensitive to the "neighbors" that are of the essence of ADHD. In ADHD, these neighboring control circuits 1) for cognitive control and 2) for social-emotional control develop later than motor control; and not only because motor system develops alongside these, but starting and reaching its mature plateau earlier, it is also the "canary in the coal mine" of all three brain control systems.

Although the large body of research literature on ADHD can't possibly be reviewed in this chapter, one longitudinal study using repeated magnetic resonance imaging provides a particularly striking illustration of how development "lags" in children with ADHD. This NIMH study revealed a three-year delay but an eventually normal structure of the front half of the cerebral cortex, such that the children with ADHD were 10.5 years old (usually in the fifth grade) when the thicknesses of these structures equaled what their typically developing peers showed at 7.5 years (usually second grade). Since many elementary schools end with fifth grade, it is a dramatic finding to ponder, since the challenges of middle or junior high schools seem formidable in relation to a brain just then equaling that of the end of second grade.

The circuit for cognitive control has been popularized over the past 30 years or so under the term "executive function." It is still somewhat controversial to say that executive dysfunction is associated with ADHD; this is discussed in the chapter devoted to executive function (EF) and dysfunction (EDF). Nevertheless, ADHD presents to my clinic, concerned with academic achievement, with a relevant cognitive deficit (my term for a "processing deficit," which is pretty vague) in the domain of executive function (cognitive control). One of the problems faced by the clinician when the referring question is, "Does this child or adolescent have ADHD?" is that many of them don't meet quite the classic criteria for ADHD but have many of its dimensions and characteristics. On direct examination or even on a rating scale designed to address executive function, they do show executive *dys*function.

The analogy between "frontal lobe syndrome" and ADHD was first pointed out 30 years ago and became the starting point for a widespread search for other signs of "frontal lobe dysfunction," which in many cases are expressed as impairments in the domain of executive function (cognitive control). The developmental trio of motor control, cognitive control, and emotional control implicates circuits that represent the three major subdivisions with the frontal lobe: the motor and premotor cortex, the enormous dorsolateral prefrontal cortex for cognitive control, and the midline and underneath (lower surface) parts of the frontal lobe governing social-emotional control; the third part includes the connections (up and down) of the reward circuits and the negative (fear, anxiety) circuits. Even before neuroimaging, executive dysfunction was expected to implicate the frontal lobe and be the major characteristic of children with ADHD when it came to its impact on their academic achievement. Those who don't quite "make it" into the ADHD category, but come close to it, or may have matured into a more subtle residual state, may still show impairments of executive function.

Of course, the picture is even further complicated; lots of neuropsychiatric conditions, not only ADHD, impair executive function, among them clearly anxiety and possibly depression. Emotional life, because of its impact on various neurotransmitters, can indirectly impair the functions of the dorsolateral prefrontal cortex that are so important for the cognitive control aspect of executive function. Recently, researchers have begun to talk about the dorsolateral prefrontal cortex cognitive controls as being "cool" executive function and the aspects I refer to as social-emotional (involving the middle and under surfaces of the frontal lobes) as being "hot" executive function. The "hot" type is clearly implicated in the impulsiveness/disinhibition of ADHD.

It is beyond the scope of this chapter to delve into the many underlying brain conditions that may manifest as the syndrome of ADHD, but one association is particularly interesting; the one I have studied as a researcher and seen as a clinician is Tourette Syndrome, the disorder of multiple tics. Over half of the children with Tourette Syndrome also have ADHD, which can be their main problem before they ever have a tic and persist to be their main problem in life, as some cases of Tourette are relatively mild (not like the most dramatic ones favored by television hospital shows) with tics experienced as nuisances but not life-altering. The ADHD in such mild cases of Tourette Syndrome is much the same as in the "garden-variety" ADHD of unknown cause.

Fascinating is that in the robust minority (perhaps 40 percent) of children and teenagers with Tourette Syndrome without ADHD there are tics that may be variably troublesome, waxing and waning over time in the lifespan, but motor and cognitive abilities tend towards the superior!

Most of the children who are referred for academic underachievement have as younger children shown more of the classic full-blown characteristics of ADHD, but many of them no longer at school age or after the age of eight show numbers of symptoms required to put them over the threshold for the diagnosis. Residual or lingering problems with control functions (even outside of academic settings) reveal to clinical judgment a profile close to the classic diagnosis, although in my research I would not be able to put them into a study of ADHD. This is part of the problem with the research literature; it may not be representative of the number of people who remain close to the diagnosis of ADHD and may have more significant executive dysfunction than those who meet the clinical diagnosis. Being a clinician/researcher, I've been forced to make very precise above-threshold diagnoses for research purposes, but clinically relevant to academic achievement I've seen much executive dysfunction short of an ADHD diagnosis. (Unless you control for such things as the age, the gender or sex, the IQ, and the nature of the executive function test, you really cannot feel very satisfied by the research literature in which there is no confirmation of the executive dysfunction of children with the "above threshold" ADHD diagnosis.) What you see clinically is that children show executive dysfunction in different domains, often in the domain where their own abilities or talents are weak and they need to compensate using executive function; they are not able to achieve on the basis of "raw natural talent." For example, a person who is somewhat weak in language ability as part of their natural cognitive profile needs strong executive function to compensate. On the other hand, a great deal of raw talent or ability can mask executive dysfunction in research studies; when someone scores "average" on a verbally based executive function test because of high verbal ability the research shows "no significant impairment." In a clinical report, one can explain the profile, saying "for a person with such an excellent vocabulary, this person has only an average word output per minute and has fluency trouble only when asked to follow an exclusion rule, to filter out words that begin in a capitalized fashion (proper nouns)." The rule-breaks will be only a subscore; the total words score will look good.

Perceptual tests in general tend to bring out executive dysfunction more than language-based tasks, because language-based tasks are practiced, habitual, and do not present as much novelty or demand as much immediate orientation to an approach. Two of the tests I use in my clinic often are untimed and multiple choice, preferred because they test aspects of visual perception without requiring a motor response; but, on the other hand, they are so odd and unusual in their format that children with executive dysfunction will frequently "flunk" the test because of executive dysfunction, not poor perceptual function. Tasks involving a direct output, such as copying a complex figure, are often very good clinically for determining that there is a lack of a good plan or approach to organization, but these are very sensitive also to cases in which motor function is a problem. (Any test, no matter what it's named, rarely measures just one thing.) Contexts and contrasts are necessary in order to come to a conclusion that there is/isn't significant executive dysfunction.

Another problem in testing for executive function is that a structured one-on-one examination (an examiner is providing instructions and feedback) may "bleach out" the executive demands that would be salient when the individual would have to operate either in a group (which means essentially resisting distraction by the group) or alone, being able to generate approaches to tasks, keep the instructions in working memory, and sustain a plan. Most people "look better" on a battery of executive function tasks than they would look with similar demands either alone doing their homework or in the classroom doing work at their seats. Again, you don't necessarily see the executive dysfunction in very intellectually gifted children in elementary school, because the demands are structured for them, demands that don't reach a level that taxes their executive function, especially if they happen to be gifted in the language-based abilities most important in the elementary school years. Middle school, high school, and college represent increasing stepwise incremental demands for independent functioning, often expressed as "taking responsibility for your own work," including organization, time management, and task planning.

The clinical fact of executive dysfunction is often complicated by coexisting anxiety, much more common in my clinic than depression. There has been an increase in academic competitiveness, the emphasis on high-stakes testing, the "straight and narrow" accelerated curriculum in many schools in so-called "good school districts." Over the past several years, this has led to an increase in the general level of anxiety surrounding anything school related. The problem is that anxiety alone can completely simulate the executive dysfunction of ADHD that evidence supports is more neurodevelopmentally based; I've had to use lots of other facts to distinguish ADHD from anxiety, factoring in the early and preschool history as well as the motor exam in the prepubertal children; developmental history and the motor exam will help to pinpoint "brain factors operating here," even if there is a coexisting overlay of anxiety. Children with learning disabilities (LD) will often become anxious, which is mistaken for showing signs of ADHD. Even more of a complication is that those with ADHD may also suffer from anxiety, in which case both must be taken into consideration when creating a treatment plan.

Parents will ask to what extent medication will be helpful if the child doesn't quite reach the threshold for a classic diagnosis of ADHD of any type. The answer is usually surprising to them because, while not a "cure-all," the medication is often very helpful independent of any diagnosis in dealing with at least the "basic step" of attention allocation, which is based on inhibition.

This is because the apparent double negative (seemingly contradictory) "stimulating inhibition" is probably the most robust effect of the stimulant medications. Of course, the stimulant medications don't just go to one target in the brain; we hope the stimulants substantially arrive at and enhance the most high-level part of the brain, the command center responsible for inhibition, both socially and cognitively. Inhibition cognitively is absolutely necessary for allocating attention to tasks that we are demanded to do, because we always have competing, more attractive things to do. (It also appears that the number of ubiquitous attractive things with screens in the lives of school-age children and adolescents have escalated over the 48 years I've been seeing such an age group. The ability to think and implement, "No, I will not text my friends or go on Facebook" when these pieces of equipment are so readily at hand is an example of the increased need to inhibit in order to allocate attentional resources to schoolwork. Perhaps these devices have contributed to the apparent increase in those meeting criteria for ADHD.)

There is much less evidence that the more mature executive functions, those involving organization, time management and planning (OTMP) are significantly impacted by medication. Coaching for OTMP has become more popular, although not yet enshrined in any school programs as part of a remedial plan. The existing 504 Plans that come under the Federal Law (a law more recent than 94–142) for inclusion of students with "disabilities" are based on a quite outmoded concept that ADHD or ADD are "disorders of limited alertness" and refer mainly to where the child is seated (in the classroom close to the teacher for the teacher to keep reminding them, perhaps" alerting" them, to pay attention) or seated in a quiet, completely separate room where it is felt that there are few "distractions." These 504 items express a contradictory and inconsistent view, since being alone in a separate room could be argued to actually decrease your arousal/alertness and allow the internal distraction of "mind wandering." There is no Individualized Educational Plan (IEP) for "executive coaching," although the word "organization" is used in IEPs (under PL 94–142) for those children who do have a demonstrable academic skills-defined learning disability, help for which can be incorporated into conventional IEPs. But if a child does not have a demonstrable "official" learning disability (e.g., in reading) listed in the codes of the state versions of public laws on special education, then there is no defined school responsibility for remedial executive (OTMP) coaching. There are some research studies on executive coaching with, again, conflicting and contradictory results attributable to sample differences depending on the age, gender, and IQ of the child, training of the coaches, and the duration and specific ingredients of the executive coaching.

At the present time, it is clinically important to emphasize a multimodal (many-sided) approach to a child who appears to either fit (or come close to fitting) the diagnosis of ADHD, a child with immature cognitive controls by history and demonstrable executive dysfunction on evaluation. It stands to reason that the evaluation cannot be shortened very much without losing all of the information co-factors and contrasts ("how strong are you here" or "how weak are you there") when analyzing how the executive aspects of a task relate to the nonexecutive cognitive abilities or talents' deficits. The minimum time I have found that makes it possible to evaluate a child over the age of seven is three hours, with a necessity for four hours if we are dealing with high school students. The multimodal program to help those with ADHD can be generated after the evaluation; in my clinic, medication is the final item discussed, preceded by school placement, special educational intervention, parent training and counselling in behavior management and emotional support, and sometimes individual psychotherapy for the child or teenager.

There are important differences between boys and girls with ADHD, both on direct assessment of functions and on imaging of the brains. I've been among those performing research focusing on girls with ADHD. My overview is that the girls are referred at later ages than the boys, have more motor immaturity relative to typical girls than is the case with boys, seem more predominantly inattentive and "day-dreamy," yet have more serious social-emotional control and hence adjustment difficulties than do boys with ADHD. (Brain imaging also shows more of the social-emotional control centers, midline and underneath parts of the frontal lobe, smaller than typical in girls with ADHD relative to the degree of diminution in boys with ADHD.)

Having explained the executive dysfunction concept, I now turn to its impact on the social aspects of life, problematic even with those not quite above-threshold for ADHD or residual when older. With failing "baby steps" within the "hot" or social executive domain, many children experience exclusion and rejection and thus gradually are socially deprived, analogous to those who have been educationally deprived. (A learning disability is difficult to diagnose if there is educational deprivation.) Annoying or aggressive preschoolers are not invited or welcome at social experiences. In other words, if a child starting even as young as age three is an annoying child, a child who "gets in your face," or who cries, who hits, or who displays in any way unacceptable expressions of disinhibited emotion, aggression, or disruption, that child is likely to fail to make friends in school or teams, to be gradually excluded from lists of invitees to play dates or birthday parties. Without intervention, they may gradually be deprived of learning situations for social executive function. The special characteristics that are captured by the term "hot" with respect to social adjustment are like this: when a person's emotions are aroused while emotional expression is not inhibited, it tends to make it impossible (or at least very difficult) to process the reactions of others for negative feedback, especially nonverbal, such as "rolling of eyes" or body postures of withdrawal. In other words, trying to process the reaction of another person in a social interchange once your own emotions are aroused and expressed is like trying to see to drive in a thunderstorm; it is hard to see through the obscured "windshield" of your own anger, tears, or frustration. You are not able to do what Dr. Russell Barkley calls "separation of affect," which is a synonym for "inhibit your own emotional expressivity," to "talk yourself down," or "count to ten," so as to be able to process reactions and learn from the consequences of your loss of self-control.

Treatment programs for ADHD or not-quite-ADHD are multimodal. Although stimulant medication is the most well-publicized, it is only a fraction of an intervention program. My summary is that medication is "neither cure nor curse." My clinic colleague, special educator and gifted observer Carol Gross, says, "stimulant medication makes the student reachable and teachable." Since teaching of adaptive behavior goes on at home and in the community as well as in school, "reachable and teachable" is a desirable general goal, but each individual profile will suggest when and where (school only, for sports, lessons, and religious activities?) medication might be recommended and given a trial. As a clinician, I regard the treatment with stimulant medication as a prime example of "the art of medication," meaning that it is tailored to the specific needs at a given age and with individual life demands, ever flexible and ready to change with the concerns of the patient or the parents of the patient. (The starting point is always evidence-based, although there is no correct starting or eventually effective dose, only "start low and increase slowly" for each individual, titrating the dose to achieve the desired benefit but always limited by any side effect experienced by that individual: the "art" comes in when treating each patient as an individual at a specific time.)

As for side effects of stimulants, these are blessedly observable, not requiring blood tests. The side effects are often transient, such as headaches at the beginning of use. The other side effects are handled by changes of dose, timing of doses, and for appetite suppression possessing the wonderful characteristic that the medication may be taken *after eating*. Working with the family during the first few weeks of prescribing medication will usually be sufficient to deal with these issues.

What is the rest of the multimodal program? First of all, but most difficult to find, is behavior modification of the modern, positively oriented variety. Such behavioral management therapy, *both home and school*, is the best proven way to teach adaptive behavior to the children we are considering in this chapter. Educational help in the form of executive coaching is also usually beneficial but might require private (outside of school) resources. Counselling or psychological therapy may be required in those cases in which emotional problems, most often anxiety, have become "layered" on top of the basic ADHD-associated symptoms. Most important of all is an attitude of good-natured warmth, expectation of growth, acceptance of immaturity, poised to be positively reinforcing, yet clear and firm in providing structure. (An enjoyment of children and a sense of humor wouldn't hurt, either.)

9

Dyslexia

Forty-five years ago, the leading question (when nobody had heard of the term Attention Deficit Hyperactivity Disorder) people often asked in my clinic was "Does my child have dyslexia or does my child have a language disorder of a broader nature?" With the increasing use of the term ADHD and with the increasing spread of the diagnosis given great scope by the term "Autistic Spectrum Disorder," language disorders as the context for reading problems have become much less frequently spoken about or thought of then was the case 40 years ago. The older way of thinking of dyslexia as the very mildest form of language disorder is closer to the neurobiological reality, because in fact dyslexia actually means "trouble with words" (one's lexicon is one's dictionary of words); dyslexia is a particular circumscribed form of a language disorder. In its purest form, dyslexia refers to problems with the speech sound level of language.

Think of language as being in a kind of a pyramid or an iceberg, with the broadest base the pragmatic, which means adjusting to the social context to communicate, the next level being semantics (meaningful words), the level above that being syntax/grammar (which also bears some smaller burden of meaning, the connections and specifications of words) and the top but narrowest level of the pyramid being speech sounds, often referred to as the "phonology." In other words, the broad base of language is in its communicative function between people, that is, its social interactive function, then above that is a layer of the meanings of words, both as we receive them and as we express them (these being the portion of the iceberg that is huge but beneath the surface of the water). The level above that is the syntactic sentence structures or relational words that link how words in a language of different types like nouns, verbs, prepositions, and so forth relate to each other, and the most rarified and in a sense abstract yet superficial level being that of the speech sounds themselves. One can think of dyslexia as a disorder that represents difficulty with the "tip of the iceberg." Think of that pyramid as an iceberg with just a little tip showing above the water, the "speech sound" or phonology tip. Of course, this is an oversimplification just for the purposes of making a diagram about the relationship of dyslexia to the rest of language disorder syndromes, but it is as close to our understanding as is currently available from a considerable amount of clinical and research experience concerning learning how to read.

School personnel, both psychologists and teachers, prefer to refer to dyslexia as "reading disability." In fact, in the official

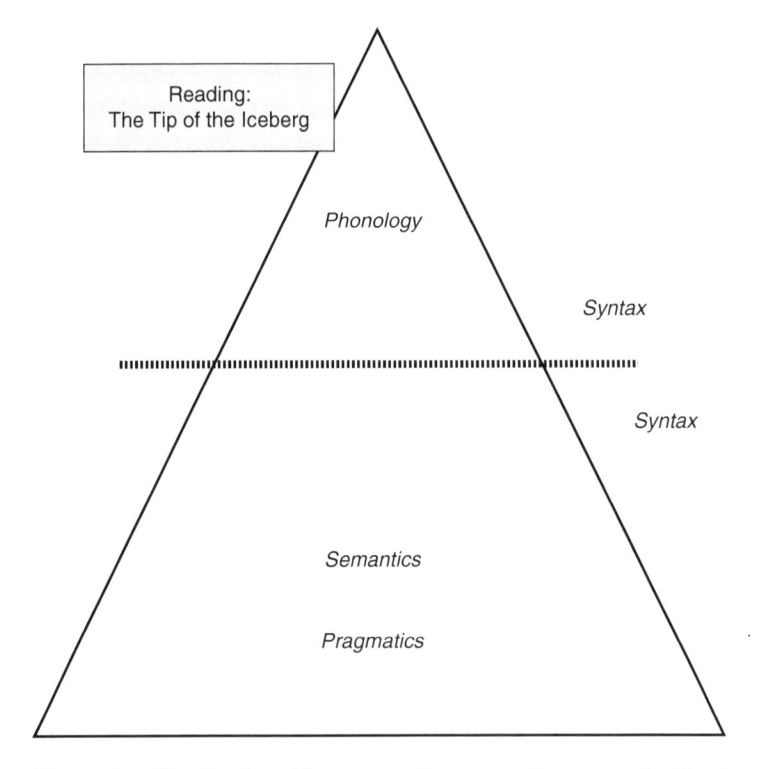

Figure 9.1 The levels of language, from most communicative to most speech specific.

DSM-5, the diagnostic code is "specific reading disability" and the word "dyslexia" does not appear. The word "dyslexia" does appear in the neurological literature and in the research literature, often preceded by "developmental" when talking about children, because without that modifier the dyslexia might be something that was a consequence of a stroke or other insult or injury to the brain in a literate adult, long after the period of rapid early development of the brain and acquisition of skills.

The purest dyslexic is a person who is not delayed in development of speech and language milestones, has a good vocabulary, scores very well on language tests involving both receptive and expressive language, and has a robust verbal IQ as well as other aspects of IQ. Yet that person appears to have difficulty when encountering the task of learning how to read. Sometimes, in fact, by virtue of learning whole words in a memorized way, the very verbally well-endowed and memory well-endowed child will not really seem to be "dyslexic" until one takes into account 1) the speed of reading and 2) ability to "crack the code" and acquire new words. (Memorizing them by sight is a formidable task compared with using the tools of the alphabetic principle with which to encounter and unlock new words. Certainly when the process of written language involves spelling and writing words, whole word memorization is a relatively inefficient tool and slows the child down considerably in the early grades. The English language is so irregular, however, that many words must be spelled by memorization; my favorite examples are all the words containing "-ough." The other sense of the word "slow" (beyond the slow early acquisition of sight words) applies to the lifelong rate of reading, which appears to be less rapid when one follows the whole word semantic route, seemingly going straight to meaning.

Even reading silently, research has shown, cannot bypass in the brain the network for the process of connecting the written whole word to its meaning, functional magnetic imaging activation studies show that even expert readers are evoking a spoken equivalent of a written word in the speech programming area of the brain (but not going on to activate the muscles for speech output), then connecting inner speech to the meaning of the word. Nonfluent reading out loud is another hint that the person who is using the whole word memorization approach is not optimally using the alphabetic principle; oral reading fluency is slowed down even without the added factor of unfamiliar words having to be encountered and memorized. (Reading languages like Chinese that do not use the alphabetic principle is entirely based upon "sight words," a formidable memory load.)

The person with pure dyslexia is a person underendowed with a talent for speech sounds, what boils down to a "tin ear for language." I think there is a direct analogy to a person who is not well endowed for musical activities, who has a "tin ear for music." The life history of such a person tends to make this very clear because the usual way foreign language is taught in school is not effective for students with a history of dyslexia. If placed into an immersion situation, especially if there is true practical necessity for learning the language, then the "untalented" may approach the success there has been in learning the native language. The reason a person with dyslexia often has tremendous difficulty learning how to speak a foreign language is that it is another challenge to phonology, to producing and attaching a new set of speech sounds to older concepts. There is often no delay in acquisition of the primary "real world" language for the child with the most specific or pure dyslexia, because the speech sounds that have to be correlated with meaningful words in real life are enveloped in a multisensory set of associations, including powerful pragmatics of having their needs met and relationships formed. Learning a second language in exactly the same way, by being thrown into or immersed in a "real world" situation, allows the same heavily motivated and reinforced association network to facilitate learning the phonology of the foreign language. In the classroom, however, there is usually a word-on-word tacking on of the foreign word to the previously learned English word, making it more like reading than like speaking, piling code upon code, analogous to the visual-to-auditory decoding for reading.

There is a gray zone in terms of how strong oral language really is for people who are called purely dyslexic. Repeatedly in a clinical evaluation one finds that such individuals have apparently not quite grasped the exact speech sounds or the sequence of speech sounds in polysyllabic low frequency words or words that are not common, habitual, or acquired outside of the academic context. In other words, again the "tin ear for language" asserts itself when the child is tested on a picture naming test and comes out with substitutions of speech sounds or mis-sequencing of sounds in the more lengthy or lower frequency words. This does not usually result in real life in an impoverished vocabulary, but it is a tell-tale sign of a person having a weak phonological aptitude. Sometimes what such people say appear to be amusing "Malapropisms." Sometimes they say such things as "tunnel" for "funnel" when confronted with a picture of a "funnel" on the Boston Naming Test, which is a picture naming challenge. Another example would be the inability to retrieve the word at all but the ability to explain that the very same unretrieved word could have another meaning! This has happened repeatedly on the Boston Naming Test in my clinic when children look at the picture of the sort of compass used for drawing a circle and look at me and say, "I can't think of the word, but it is also the word for what you use to tell where the north is when you are lost in the woods." This is a very clear demonstration of high semantic competence coexisting with an inability to retrieve the precise sequence of speech sounds that makes up the name. It is as though the shadow of the word exists in a semantic network, not well connected with the speech sounds.

On critical evaluation, if one uses a sensitive test like a picture naming test, one can pick up some expressive language characteristics of the "pure dyslexic" that betray imprecision of the phonological (speech sound) component of linguistic competence. On IQ testing and even on many full languages batteries, there is no challenge of that precise nature (like the Boston Naming Test) that will bring out speech sound difficulty, which can be subtle. This is why it is best to remember that dyslexia belongs by its very meaning ("trouble with words") to the general category or spectrum of language disorders. This fact has been very much left in the shadows recently. However, 40 years ago the context was better appreciated, since it was well recognized that there was a very strong probability that a child who did present with a language disorder in the preschool years of life would go on to have some trouble with reading. This would be true even if the receptive language appeared to be perfect, again the association of the speech sounds with real world associations was not impaired, but precision in expressive language or speech sound production at a more "endpoint" level was impaired.

It is still not completely clearly understood how the different possible "way stations" along the circuit from the posterior to anterior path of the language network of the brain can impair what the speech pathologist refers to as "phonology." Obviously, it sometimes is at the level of perceptual difficulty because in severe instances, there will be receptive as well as expressive language disorder. However, it is far more common that receptive language is relatively intact while somewhere along the pathway to the speech programming area there will be some kind of weak connection or lack of sufficient quantitative ability to convey the message, or there may be something inadequate at the pre-production step, which is a motor speech programming area. Even to this day we do not really know how to "parse" the segments of this pathway.

The "big picture" to keep in mind about early reading is that it is essentially a "see it/say it" transaction. The saying is very much involved in the positive learning. Those of us who consider ourselves fluent, rapid, and completely comfortable readers silently do not realize that imaging has clearly shown that even in adult highly competent readers, those with no consciousness of speech going on in the mind, the speech area is always activated during the time of silent fluid reading. In other words, the brain is always going "I see it, I say it" even though the "saying it" has "gone underground" (not connected to oral movement) many years before.

Having talked about dyslexia as a very subtle disorder placed within the context of a language disorder, I would like to review the classical "roadmap" of the human brain in terms of the language system. Although this is derived from the adult, it is a system that is the eventual model to be attained by the developing brain. We'll be talking about right-handed persons and the vast majority of left-handed persons whose language is lateralized predominantly to the left side of the brain. The language circuit itself consists of an auditory association area in the temporal lobe called Wernicke's area, a connection between the two ends by means of a bundle referred to as the Superior Longitudinal Fasciculus, a crucial portion of which is the arcuate because it arches as it goes up from the temporal to the parietal lobe, and at the front end the speech programming area called Broca's area. There are also connections into this language system and out of this language system with a visual association area that is behind it at the junction of the occipital and temporal lobes and most importantly in reciprocal connections with a very important major association area that gathers input from all three major senses. To make visual to speech sound connections is critical for reading at the decoding stage. To connect the speech sounds with the meanings, the semantics, depends upon the association area that integrates all the sensory information (except taste and smell). In the context of adult acquired disorders, much of which is handed down to us from the nineteenth-century study of people with "strokes" (meaning that blood supply has been blocked in some way and caused damage to selected areas of the brain), we know that there are several language disorders (aphasias) complicated by "alexia" that are caused by damage to the areas in the left hemisphere language areas or to the connections between them, and to the higher order multisensory association area. We also know that anything that disconnects the visual association area from the language circuits will cause a selective "dyslexia." That kind of "dyslexia," when it is acquired, is "pure" without any "dysgraphia" (spelling or writing problem). This does not apply directly to children because children haven't yet learned all of the spelling patterns and made associations with all the other sensory modalities or between the spelling patterns and the motor ability to write them, so you don't see pure dyslexia without dysgraphia in children.

Now it's important to jump back and consider the nature of what is a "phoneme" or a "speech sound" unit when it is abstracted from meaning. The "phoneme," contrary to popular terminology, is not an "auditory" unit. (I will say more later about what's unsatisfactory about talking about "auditory processing" in such a broad brush manner). The "phoneme" is built out of a correspondence between an auditory speech sound perception and a mouth position as programmed (even if it is silently) in Broca's area, the speech programming area. By analogy to basic chemistry, just as water is neither "H" nor "O" but is "H_2O," so a phoneme is "speech sound perception blended with speech sound production programming." We do not yet know with the precision we know about water what the ratio or proportion of "speech sound perception" to "speech motor program" might be; for many years I have very much wanted somebody to do some research on the capacity to be "phonologically aware" or use phonics to acquire basic reading skill in children whose cerebral palsy affects their speech motor system. However, at the present time I really don't have data on this in order to be able to talk about the "ratio," but want to firmly go on record stating that we cannot really continue to talk about the foundation for the use of phonics in reading as "auditory processing" not further specified.

"Auditory" is a very big term. There are auditory association areas on both sides of the brain. Again, sticking to what we know best, the majority brain organization seen in right-handed people and the vast majority of nonright-handed people, the left side of the brain has what we have called the temporal plane, which is a very large flat area (formal name *planum temporale*) on the top surface of the temporal lobe, right next to the receiving area for hearing, the primary auditory input; it is a very large territory of speech sound processing, usually ten times bigger than its "mate" (like the other glove in a pair of gloves) on the right side. Importantly, on the right side of the brain the homologous region, the right temporal plane, is an auditory processing area with three "mandates," not all of them equal "talents" in different individuals. The most familiar "variable talent" in the auditory processing of the right side of the brain is that involving musical pitch. The second is environmental sounds/noises perception (recently getting more complex with the different "notification" sounds on our digital devices). The third is the perception that allows the discrimination of the emotional state or intentional attitude of a person speaking to us, called "emotional prosody." In other words, on the right, crowded into a temporal plane that is usually only *one-tenth* the size of the one on the left (devoted to speech sounds), are three kinds of auditory processing systems, musical, environmental sound discriminations, and emotional (tones of voice) processing. Clearly, it is not accurate and it could even be harmful for someone doing an assessment for school purposes who has given a phonological speech sound test, important for school but not the entire auditory domain, to announce to the parents that the child has an impairment in "auditory processing." While strictly relevant within the boundaries of the educational assessment, this might actually be prejudicial to the parents' understanding of the child. For example, the child might be a potentially great musician! Precision of vocabulary is therefore not just a matter of being a "language Nazi" or a language police person; it is a question of rendering a "real-world" accurate profile of a child to the child's parents.

When the child or adolescent comes to the clinic with the question being whether he or she "has dyslexia," the reading scores and IQ measurements will in all probability have been done and some collection of report cards forwarded, so in the specialty clinic, the issue will be to try to collect evidence of "intrinsic" fundamental brain characteristics of developmental dyslexia. First, there should be a neurologically based language examination (please see chapter on language disorders for why this is necessary and is not synonymous with verbal IQ) to establish the context of the reading problem. (Remember the "iceberg" metaphor; we need to explore the broader, deeper language competencies "below the surface.")

The establishing evidence for dyslexia is confirmed by subtle but not disordered findings in the language evaluation that will yield important aspects of the recommendations for intervention. The compelling evidence comes from two fundamental challenges, as described and elaborated by Marianne Wolf (with whose doctoral dissertation I had the honor to be involved) and her colleagues; this is the Double Deficit scheme of dyslexia, the severe type showing both deficits and the more moderate types showing only one or the other: 1) phonological awareness is tested and 2) Rapid Automatized Naming (RAN) is tested. Both challenges can be given as early as four years of age; the former is tapped in many different available assessment tools, with the latter being available either as a "stand alone" or incorporated as a subtest into other assessment instruments labeled as devoted to phonological processing. (It is still argued by some experts that RAN is but one component of phonological processing, but I, as the originator of this assessment, as well as the collaborator with two generations of my trainees, have much data indicating its separate significance: most compelling is the use of RAN in China to predict dyslexia in these nonalphabetic written language learners.)

2	6	9	4	7	6	2	9	7	4
9	4	2	7	4	2	6	7	9	6
6	2	9	7	9	4	7	2	4	6
4	6	7	2	4	9	6	9	2	7
9	2	4	7	6	7	2	6	4	9

Time [ ]   Errors [ ]   Self-Corrections [ ]

Figure 9.2 Number page of RAN (the others are colors, letters, and, for preschool, objects); the task is to name the 50 items of the page as quickly as possible.

Although there is relatively satisfactory understanding of the ways in which "an inconvenient brain" may underlie dyslexia, there are at present very general, not so individualized, principles to guide intervention. Provide help early. Maximize instruction time in terms of frequency, amount of time per day (not exceeding a half hour to start with, to avoid exhaustion and frustration, if starting early in elementary school). Keep up the intervention for several years, gradually "weaning" and transitioning to support for written expression. Be sure there is a qualified teacher/tutor using a proven remedial program. Controversy still exists as to whether the sessions have to be individual or in a small group; this may be resolved by seeing how the personality or emotional tendencies of the child allow for the small (five or fewer) group. Recently, a highly regarded private special school devoted to learning disabilities has moved to some individual sessions sooner when progress in small groups is stalled.

The essential elements, shared by all proven programs, are that instruction should be direct, systematic, and should be at least substantially based on what we call the alphabetic principle, the use of phonics to "sound out" (some say using phonics to "attack") new words. More variable is the devotion of some portion of each session to sight words, sometimes derived from the phonics exercise plus the irregular (dare one say "irrational") words that abound in English. (The admirable richness of the English language carries with it the "price tag" of spellings imported from several languages and then further modified by usage.)

Later on—how much later is a function of how well the basic skills are progressing—irregular word spelling is introduced. (Please see chapter on motor skills for the obstacles caused by handwriting.)

Fluency training, comprehension training, vocabulary building, and enriched language experiences both with books read to the child or with audiobooks, are important surrounding contributors to successful reading remediation/intervention. It is important that we not become rigid in commitment to the best method, allowing compensations and idiosyncratic ways of working around the written words to reach comprehension.

All evidence-based interventions share structured approaches involving small steps, with reinforcement of learned skills and with an emphasis on making the basic procedures automatic. These programs do not favor memorized chants of "rules" but foster applied practice of the procedures.

When mature enough to be available, children are encouraged to articulate their own individual strategies ("metacognition") for decoding and comprehending text. Some of these evidence-based interventions will be described in the websites listed after the References.

What is to be avoided is recourse to "easy answers" or superficially reasonable interventions, like vision therapies or computer programs that make extravagant claims to "fix the brain" in some fundamental and permanent fashion that makes specialized teaching of reading unnecessary. These will be discussed in the chapter on neuromythology; unsubstantiated interventions arise as consequences of unsubstantiated theories of the causes of dyslexia.

10

Math and Miscellaneous Learning Disabilities

The biological basis for mathematics is present in many living creatures other than human beings, making mathematics very different from reading and writing (that even for human beings can be regarded as "unnatural acts" or cultural artifacts). Many vertebrates, even fish and frogs, display behaviors that signify some kind of number sense, because their decisions show ability to "count" or respond to greater or lesser number sets; described by terms like "numerosity" or "subitizing," number sense is a deeply embedded ability across many species, mammals and birds included, and is considered to be conserved for its useful survival properties. Fish are able to "count," in that guppies will gravitate towards swimming with larger schools of fish rather than smaller ones; a frog can count how many noises its rivals are making in a mating situation and will try to outmatch the mating calls up to the number seven. (Amazingly, spiders have been found to actually count up their "savings" by number rather than the total mass of accumulated prey caught in their webs!) Some animals in fact appear to be able to make discriminations between groups of numbers up to ten, although it is more difficult if the groups differ by only one or two and are easier for the birds and mammals to discriminate if the difference within the first nine total numbers are at least three items apart. Chimpanzees are able to learn to associate actual Arabic numerals with a number of items, up to the Arabic numeral "9." They can arrange the Arabic numerals as well as the groups of items in ascending order from the least to the most! In fact, chimpanzees have been found to have better working memory for numbers than human beings do, showing the ability to remember the locations of numerals that have been presented to them in a random sprinkled array after a delay when blank boxes come up for them to tap. (It is thought that some of this wonderful visually based working memory has been preempted or repurposed for language in human beings, and it can be argued that what we have gained is more important than what we have lost in terms of this working memory for spatial arrays of numerals.)

It is also the case that those who study human languages have found that the linguistic words for the numbers one through five are very similar across many different languages and when tracked across generations seem to change less than other words in the language. Thus, both across many species of living things and in terms of human linguistic usage it can be said that numbers and their associated representations are highly conserved aspects of biology in the brain. (The frog accomplishments referred to above actually have been found to be based upon certain neurons in the midbrain that make it possible to count and have been referred to as the "midbrain neuroabacus.")

Truly specific mathematics LD (MLD) has been reported clinically to be associated with poor performances on tests of visual perception and visual memory, but in that form is very rare. Much more common is the kind of MLD that is associated with the use of the number symbols and the number words used in counting and in representing numbers. This is why there is much in common with the language-based learning disability we call "dyslexia" in most cases. If the linguistic component that is involved in counting items and memorizing math facts and the meaning of specific numerals in the language system are acquired, then even those who are perceptually poorly endowed are able to use language to compensate at an adequate, if not optimal, level. Some degree of difficulty appreciating the spatial nature of the notation, the place value of number (certainly a visual-spatial construct) precludes being "good at math," and this compensation is achieved at the expense of speed. Math fluency, the speed with which calculations, beyond rote number facts, can be accomplished for numbers of more than one digit, is slowed down if the immediate visual-spatial perception and "the mind's eye" variety of working memory are weak. In other words, the compensation by the linguistic component usually serves to at least get a child a "passing grade" in basic arithmetic, although the child will not be fast or fluent doing multidigit calculations and will certainly not excel at "doing calculations mentally" (which requires "a mind's eye" or visualization). Few such children actually fail or are identified as falling several grade levels behind in math, but they "pass" while being slow and plodding. Even geometry in high school may be "passed" by those who use verbal logical approaches to this obviously visual-spatial form of mathematics. Algebra is more amenable to language mastery, as it is basically "naked syntax," rigid grammatical manipulations without nouns; as long as slowness is tolerated, high school mathematics short of calculus can be mastered without much visual-spatial ability. (To be gifted in mathematics requires an integrated trio of visual-spatial, verbal, and executive abilities; but this is not to be confused with what it takes to be a student who passes or even attains "B" grades in mathematics.)

Far more commonly found in recent research on MLD is the major role played by executive function in successful acquisition and production of arithmetic and higher mathematical skills like algebra. This is because many procedures have to be followed, requiring both planning across time and organizing across space. Perhaps the most dramatic arithmetical example of the role of executive function comes when we look at long division. In that particular arithmetical operation, there is an "educated guess" followed by a hypothesis-testing step in which the number chosen has to be validated by another step using math facts elicited from stored-up memory. There is also a spatial component of shifting columns vertically as one writes down the successive steps in a long division problem. Clearly also requiring executive function is the solution of word problems, because the numbers involved have to be extracted from the frequently complex conditional sentences; analysis and synthesis has to be performed in order to solve a word problem without getting lost in the particulars of the "verbiage." Finally, some word or words for the items or units of measurement in the answer to the word problem have to be held in working memory and retrieved.

To the extent that a body of publications exists on the subject of specific MLD, the most prominent combination of cognitive weaknesses (the educator's "processing problems") would be weakness in visual-spatial skill, giving rise to a lack of a strong appreciation of number meaning based on place value and mental visualization of relationships between numbers of more than one digit, complicated by weak executive functions; these are attention to detail, planning across time, organizing across space, holding components in working memory (so that one knows what step has just been done and will not endlessly repeat it), and the advanced executive function of checking/self-monitoring.

The original influential publication about MLD was done over 30 years ago within the popularized neuropsychological work of Rourke and his associates, in which "nonverbal learning disability" was announced and popularized. Nonverbal learning disability (NVLD) is not often used or discussed in recent decades and will be addressed in another chapter later in this book. For the purposes of this chapter, however, the history of NVLD was that its "flagship" sign was MLD, surrounded by visual-perceptual deficiencies and social perceptual deficiencies. The social part of the NVLD syndrome garnered a great deal of attention but has since been overshadowed by interest in ASD. Rourke thought that NVLD involving math, social, and a broad nonverbal visual-perceptual repertoire resulted from something wrong with the association areas of the right hemisphere of the brain. The contrast between language-based LD, also referred to as verbal LD, based upon left hemisphere inadequacies, was thus symmetrically contrasted (although affecting much smaller numbers of students in terms of prevalence) with NVLD based upon right hemisphere weaknesses. For some reason, Rourke and his associates and those who have perpetuated the construct of NVLD have never talked about executive function or its basis in the frontal lobes but have kept their thinking localized further back, particularly the parietal areas of the cerebral cortex, the great posterior association areas that sit at the juncture of the three major sensory/perceptual lobes, essential for language on the left and all these other nonverbal cognitive functions on the right.

Over two decades ago, a graduate student worked with me on his doctoral dissertation that attempted a replication of the work of Rourke. This graduate student managed to go to a large number of public schools in the Baltimore area and accumulate a group of children who were receiving special education classification solely on the basis of their MLD, while considered to be progressing academically well in all other areas of the curriculum. He studied these children with many questionnaires for their parents and teachers, largely focused on documenting social problems, as well as directly evaluating them with neuropsychological tests. What he found was striking and seemed to point firmly away from any conclusion that NVLD held up as the distinctive "right hemisphere" syndrome in which the MLD was embedded. All of those students with MLD who were rated by teachers and parents as socially impaired also met criteria for ADHD and their neuropsychological testing was overwhelmingly impaired in executive function rather than in visual-spatial abilities.

This was quite a startling and somewhat surprising result, but one cannot say that it contradicted the original NVLD construct, because neither a set of interviews or questionnaires addressing the issue of ADHD nor neuropsychological tests sensitive to executive function were included in the earlier NVLD research reports sharing the starting point of MLD. In the NVLD studies there were simply no data concerning either ADHD or executive functions.

When this dissertation was completed, it reminded me that a colleague in pediatric neurology, Dr. Kytja Voeller, had been very much interested in looking into whether the NVLD construct represented a right hemisphere syndrome; she had looked at all of her clinical data to accumulate a group of children who actually had some kind of either stroke or head trauma documented to be on the right side of the brain. She wanted to see whether the right side of the brain, when damaged, was responsible for all of these nonverbal learning tasks. She found that the group with evidence of damage to the right side of the brain uniformly qualified for the diagnosis of ADHD. Members of the group also did poorly on various tests sensitive to perception of facial expression of emotion, which would be relevant to a social learning disability, and they did not score nearly as well on visual-perceptual tests as they did on language tests. Dr. Voeller commented, in a way that I have repeated many times, to the effect that the nature of the tests addressing these social and other visual-perceptual capabilities places demands for executive function on the child in a way that is not the case for the testing of verbal abilities; language skills are so much more part of daily life, practiced, and habitual, that one has to really escalate task demands in order to bring executive function to the foreground. There is an inherent inequality in the degree to which assessments represent challenges to verbal versus nonverbal cognitive abilities and the relative novelty of the visual-perceptual-spatial tasks makes executive functions crucial to success on these.

Now returning to the subject of math and its difficulties, after our brief diversion into its association with the NVLD concept, we again review that before there are words or symbols for numbers, number processing depends upon an innate approximate number system not confined to human beings. The ability across many living species to "subitize" (the rather fancy term for the ability to immediately perceive the differences between groups of numbers up to about ten) is followed by approximation. For human calculations and later higher mathematics to be implemented, there has to be a symbol system that attaches written symbols/spoken names for numbers and it has to be "ordinal," which means that the symbols can be arranged along a visualized small-to-large "number line." We also reviewed the fact that enormous territories of brain must be involved in order for even the most basic kind of arithmetic to be accomplished, with connections between right and left posterior association cortex, connecting the two sides of the brain, as well as recruiting the frontal lobes.

Most of the children seen with MLD are weak in the verbal and symbolic system, although there are rare severe cases weak in both symbolic and basic number processing. Again, two-thirds of those identified with MLD have another LD or LD-related condition such as Specific Language Impairment, dyslexia, ADHD, or anxiety; the least common coexisting condition is a more general deficiency in sense of direction, social emotional perception, and other nonverbal components of what might be called NVLD or a right-hemisphere-based impairment of "visual-spatial" processing. The true dyscalculic child lacks the basic number sense represented by "subitizing" (discriminating at a glance how small sets of items differ from each other quantitatively) and approximating within the number system. Because of the highly conserved nature of basic number sense biologically, truly isolated "dyscalculia" underlying MLD is very rare as a developmental condition in human beings of normal intelligence. In normal adults who have undergone functional imaging that reveals what is activated, "subitizing" activates the right-sided posterior part of the cortex (the parietal lobe), the same as in monkeys. The number *symbols* (numerals) activate exactly the homologous areas in the left side of the brain, the same as letters of the alphabet. This is an important point: numerals and letters activate the same language area for names in the left side of the brain.

If one looks at research on intervention for MLD, training in arithmetic will bring out certain EEG rhythms that are associated with being "on-task." Increases in arithmetic skill during the intervention or shortly thereafter correlate with less frontal and more posterior parietal activation. Giving quick answers to memorized math facts, particularly multiplication tables, is a task for the brain exactly like saying a memorized poem or prayer and activates the left side language areas. The most interesting functional imaging response to intervention is that the two sides of the brain activate in synchrony with each other much more than was the case before the training. Also, there are two components of executive function (terms for which are common ground, because they are in the vocabulary of educators and psychologists as well as of professionals in the neurosciences field), *working memory* and *processing speed*, which apply to success in math in the same way in which they apply to success in reading comprehension. Now I will describe some other miscellaneous LDs that challenge "the inconvenient brain."

How about the learning disabilities that are not covered by what has been discussed so far? In a sense, dysgraphia (that covers both motor and spelling procedures involved in writing) has been covered because it can be split into the actual mechanics of production of the symbols as letter forms, covered in the chapter on motor coordination (DMCD), and dyslexia, because spelling is the most difficult application of sound-symbol association, much more demanding of precision and of correct sequence than is the use of phonics for acquiring the skill of reading. Deeper than "dysgraphia," more fundamental than handwriting and spelling skills, there lies written expression, which depends heavily on the executive functions of working memory, planning, and organization, as well as that "finishing touch" we call "checking" or self-monitoring. There is an "official" category in education for Written Expression LD.

More recently, reading comprehension has been looked at as one of the "other" learning disabilities because the "simple view of reading" (the assumption that once decoding skills become automatic there will simply follow reading comprehension), in which view comprehension is just another component within dyslexia, has largely been disproven by research. In other words, the "simple view of reading" assumed that once one could decode or read by phonic attack or by sight words, mastering the procedure of making print into speech, it would follow "as the night follows the day" that one would comprehend. However, research undertaken by my own group and by others has demonstrated that this "simple view of reading" is simply not universally applicable. There are children who acquire all of their basic decoding skills, who can rapidly "sound out" regular words and respond to irregular words by sight, who seem stuck at this surface level, but do not match their decoding by their level of reading comprehension. The reasons for reading comprehension problems can be traced to the two great cognitive domains that have the most overriding importance for all educational attainment, language and executive function. In terms of language, vocabulary and sophisticated understanding of syntax (grammar) are necessary, as reading comprehension of more complex texts is required in all school subjects. Working memory and processing speed coordinate when adequate but when deficient interact for the reverse; these are the components of executive function that can be understood as essential to effective reading comprehension. Imagine that you are slow at sentence reading (a processing speed problem) and you also have a foreshortened working memory span. Because working memory is time-locked, if you go slowly you will not be able to maintain within the time span of your working memory enough of the text in order to "understand" what is being expressed in the text. Additionally, if your working memory span is even shorter than typical, you are in "double jeopardy" when attempting to comprehend across reasonable chunks of text.

I must refer back to the issue of how ADHD and learning disabilities relate to each other. Even without reference to the NVLD issue, when we have done research concerning ADHD in populations of young children with ADHD in the early grades (first, second, and third) we can often document that they are making perfectly adequate academic progress in all subjects; but when they return two years later they have "grown into" learning disabilities in written expression, math, and reading comprehension (in order of descending severity of underachievement). That is because of the contributions of such executive skills as working memory, processing speed, planning/organization, and self-monitoring/checking behaviors to more advanced academic achievements.

> It is useful to think of two of the most well-known "inconvenient brains" as follows: Dyslexia is probably due to a permanent structural/architectural variant of brain; ADHD is probably due to a lag/delay in brain development, but not a trivial amount of time (three years) involved in the lag and certainly an ultimately important set of functions involved.

Finally, because this chapter starts with MLD, I should address definitions of a heterogeneous group of learning disabilities, other than the best-publicized "dyslexia." The status of diagnosing or categorizing a learning disability is in something of a state of flux. In the earlier years of the public law concerning specific learning disabilities, the definition was based upon documentation of a discrepancy (about how much of a gap and on which measurements a great deal of argument went back and forth). The concept most generally accepted was that there must be a gap between some measure of cognitive ability (an IQ test or a representative component of an IQ test) and a significantly lower score on a test of one or more academic skills in order to be categorized as belonging to one or more LD groups. More recently, there has been an educational movement based on research contradicting the meaningfulness of any "discrepancy" formula because of difficulties deciding what score to accept as the IQ and which academic test score, or how much of a discrepancy between scores, should be used to determine LD status for each academic skill. The leading researchers pronounce that people should not be identified as learning disabled until appropriate expert instruction has been provided, leading to the concept of defining LD by Response to Intervention (RTI). This is a very challenging and sophisticated approach in which there are stepwise levels of intervention starting the minute a child is observed by a classroom teacher to be slipping behind in the expected rate of skill acquisition in a given subject. The problems of validity of the academic skill tests, the IQ tests, and the discrepancy calculation are well-documented; but it is also the case that RTI is "easier said than done" in terms of implementation. For example, a teacher-nominated child could be put into a small group for more intensive high quality instruction. Now the problems, no longer those of the discrepancy method, are documenting what is the evidence for high quality in the method of instruction and how highly qualified as an expert is the instructor. Furthermore, it is not clear what happens if the student in the RTI model does well, exits early, and returns to the regular class, but the next step in the academic skill sequence is again a hurdle for that previously "responsive" student. It is more obvious what happens with those who are still not doing well after the first level of intervention; they receive another ten weeks of specialized instruction, perhaps in an even smaller group, and so on in stepped-up levels of intervention. By the third level of intervention, the RTI model allows the LD categorization reserved for the "remediation-resistant."

The RTI model sounds very reasonable, indeed ideal, but, as I have stated, in the "real world" there are difficulties implementing RTI because of variation in teacher identification of the problem, sometimes because children are very good at hiding their difficulties so as to appear not to need intervention, or there are problems evaluating the evidence basis for the quality of instructional methods used, in what size group, for what length of session each day and for how many weeks' duration. Finally, most difficult of all, is the problem in RTI of measuring that elusive element, the quality of the teacher.

Outside of schools, in neurological, psychological, and neuropsychological clinics, the definition of a learning disability is less quantitative and involves a demonstrably selective or specific aspect of cognition, sometimes referred to by educators as "processing," that is impaired or deficient at a given time, and for which cognitive "process" there is evidence that it is necessary for, or at least significantly contributory to, successful academic achievement.

Here again, professionals who draw upon neuroscience and cognitive science feel most comfortable, due to a long history and a large body of research, supporting a conclusion that a student has dyslexia or reading disability; but we have much less research and much less robust data with respect to all of the other categories of learning disabilities, so we are forced to admit that we are dealing with probabilities, circumstantial risk factors, and sometimes plausible relevance.

11

Neuromythology

Although, as can be seen from my introduction to this book, I am a great believer in and participant in neuroeducation, I am also aware of the fact that there are many incomplete, misunderstood, poorly documented, and purely theoretical brain-based explanations and interventions for learning disabilities. These are enthusiastic but not evidence-supported extensions from what people think are neurological facts about the organization and the development of the brain. It is wonderful to bring into schools knowledge about the developing brain, which is the basic meaning of "neuroeducation," applied to general as well as special education. On the other hand, many longstanding or current claims that education is being supplemented, enhanced, or modified on the basis of neuroscience are either completely irrelevant or exaggerated.

I wish that the most important fact of neuroscience known by educators is that plasticity of the brain, meaning the ability to change or be modified, lasts over the entire human lifespan, although some periods, usually early ones (but not *too* early) are better than others for new learning. New learning also helps to preserve our brain function (and even its microstructure, in the form of dendritic "arborization," meaning sprouting from the surfaces of neurons) and therefore prevent or postpone cognitive decline. The second fact is that, since development of the brain is highly variable at least up to about the late 30s decade of life, there is a need to evaluate each individual in terms of what stage the person's brain is "at" rather than the chronological age the person has attained. The third fact to remember is that the brain and the environment engage in an ongoing reciprocal "duet" or "dance" in which "nature and nurture" interact, each modifying the other, for better or for worse.

I am now going to list some of the misconceptions about the brain and about learning disabilities.

1. Somehow it has come to be a piece of general misinformation that we use only 10 percent of our brains. Now that we have wonderful imaging-derived measurements of the connectivity and functioning of networks in the brain, we know that the brain never really rests and even when it is in the so-called "default" model (not driven by outside influences, not task-oriented) the brain is engaging in some kind of reflection. The brain is active during sleep. It is simply not in any way documented that the brain could ever be in a state where only 10 percent of it is "used." What is remarkable is how much more use can be demonstrated in the same brain circuits, best illustrated by the fact that more than one language can be acquired using the same language system in the left side of the brain.

2. People are "left brain dominant" or "right brain dominant" types of learners. Sometimes the left is identified with "verbal" and the right is identified with "visual" and other nonverbal perceptual learning styles and is considered to be the more "creative" hemisphere. This is an exaggeration born of enthusiasm when a lot of research was done (back when I myself was in my neurology training years) on so-called "split-brain" patients, in whom uncontrolled epilepsy was being treated by disconnecting the two sides of the brain; and to everyone's amazement, the right side of the brain on its own could demonstrate wonderful nonverbal capabilities. This enthusiastic greeting of the capabilities of the right brain somehow led to the idea that we had a whole group of people who could learn in school using right-brain approaches or "styles." Unfortunately, given the nature of what is learned in school, this is simply not possible; but it is certainly possible to bring to bear upon school learning compensatory and enhancing techniques from the nonverbal repertoire of the right brain. It is unavoidable to accept, however, that almost everything that we do in school and is required of us academically is left brain dependent. This idea of people who are "left brain learners" or "right brain learners" came out of some interesting research of how each hemisphere

supports its own special cognitive domains, but does not reflect how the connected brain (or even the immature, less-well-connected brain of the developing child) can actually function. It is an illustration of how "neuromyths" can be oversimplifications of neuroscience inaccurately applied to education. It has also generated a lot of special education and even general education recommendations based on "learning styles." Even without referring to the brain, researchers have accumulated evidence that "learning styles" do not generate effective instructional programs.

3. Consuming sugary snacks and beverages leads to hyperactivity and decreased attention span. This belief came out of some research more than three decades ago; based on clinical anecdotes, it was thought that food additives (and somehow this morphed into the sugar content of the snacks in which additives were ingredients) could cause the syndrome we call ADHD. Parents are convinced of this and many teachers agree, but there is no evidence to support this contention applied to school-age children. One of the confounding factors is that many of the contexts in which high-sugar food or drinks are consumed (think "birthday parties") are those in which excitement is high while structure and supervision may be at a minimum; and this may allow children to "regress," behaving like younger children in unleashed hyperactivity and failure to pay attention to adults. Again, there is little or no evidence for placing the blame on sugar (which has a lot of other unhealthy outcomes to account for); the few studies in support of a sugar impact report this in preschool children, but fail to account for context.

4. Teenagers have immature brains, especially the frontal lobes, in which are represented important self-control mechanisms, and thus cannot be held responsible for self-control. This is an example of leaping from "less" to "none," a maturational fact taken too far. While it is certainly a reasonable conclusion from brain studies that legal responsibilities cannot be assigned at the *adult* level to teenagers (and I would even extend adolescence to at least 25 years of age) it is taken to an extreme of exaggeration by the use of the word "can't" in front of "control themselves." What would be far more reasonable is to take a graded, noncategorical approach. Adolescents have a difficult

time controlling themselves; the hormones stimulating their emotional brains may be out of balance with reciprocal frontal connections ("hot" executive function) so that teens need more explicit, positively oriented structure from adults in order to help them to control themselves. ("Friends, Romans, countrymen, lend me your *frontal lobes*," with apologies to Shakespeare.) This is another example of assisting a developing brain with learning; this learning concerns management of emotionally stimulating situations. To go to the extreme of saying that teenagers are completely incapable of self-control or conclude that harsh negative discipline is the only option is counterproductive. Just as is the case with children with ADHD, what is effective is to look at the risks/reward balance within the model of "antecedents, behavior, consequences (ABC)" and help to both structure the antecedents (elements in the environment that would tend to reduce risk-taking) and provide a warm but firm environment in which there is encouragement ("I know you can make good decisions") and there are frequent rewards for self-control, even "baby steps" in that direction.

5. Dyslexia is characterized by reversals in reading and writing. Although reversals in reading and writing do occur in dyslexic children and probably persist somewhat longer than they do in other children, reversals are very common in the early grades in all of general education. Research I did in my years working with Rita G. Rudel at Columbia revealed that the writing samples of second graders who were progressing perfectly normally in learning how to read contained just as many letter reversals as did the writing samples of their dyslexic classmates. (This is recognized in our culture: think of the late lamented retail chain, Toys R[reversed] Us.) It proved too difficult to study large groups of children one at a time reading aloud to find out whether "was/saw" or "dog/God" would be read out loud to a greater or lesser degree in the two groups, but I must say that in my over four decades of testing reading aloud in children referred for dyslexia I have rarely heard such reversals. That there are sequencing errors of spelling in dyslexic persons, including mixed-up sequences of syllables as well as letters, is true but is not necessarily on a "visual" basis. The origins of this emphasis on visual "reversals" lie in the work of Dr. Samuel Torrey Orton who wrote (in the year that I was born) a book

about children's reading, writing, and speaking problems, in which he put forth the *hypothesis* that all of these developmental problems were due to conflict and inconsistency between the two sides of the brain; if the left side did not become supremely dominant, the results were speech and reading problems. This was thought to show up in reading as inconsistency of the direction in which all of the units of printed language were perceived. This "flip-flop" explanation for reversals was called "strephosymbolia" (meaning "twisted symbols"). Careful reading of Dr. Orton's book reveals that the reversals were not considered by him to be the sole or major source of the reading problem.

The first research project I ever did was about the perceptual reversal hypothesis in dyslexic eight-year-old children; suffice it to say that it was a "dud," a dead end. There were no dyslexic misperceptions based upon which visual field (on what side of the brain) symbols were presented; the "same/different" discrimination of directional orientation of symbols was made flawlessly within and across visual fields. Some good came out of this failure to support the reversals hypothesis. In one of the most memorable episodes of my career, one of the dyslexic children said to me after performing without any errors, "This is a stupid test!" I responded that he was undoubtedly right, because by then I had tested so many children who, like him, were dyslexic but were having no difficulty with my "twisted symbols" challenge. He then volunteered (and I will never forgive myself for failing to recall his name and use his name in order to give him credit) his insight. "My problem is not seeing whether they face the same direction, to the right or to the left when these similar looking symbols are seen together: but when I see one of them *alone*, I am not sure whether its name is 'Joe' or 'Moe'." (He actually said those alternative names. What a brilliant observation!) In other words, he did not experience a perceptual problem, there was not a "war" for directional discrimination between the two sides of the brain's visual system, but there was a lack of firm association between a symbol and its name. This emphasis on *naming* launched the most successful research of my career. I also went on to reflect on the fact that the way that the lower case "b" and the lower case "d" *sound* over the telephone is very difficult to tell apart, and could be an equal source of "reversals" coupled with their visual appearance. (Who reverses written "p" and "q"? Visually they are mirror images but their names are phonologically distinct.)

6. There is a whole group of treatments for dyslexia that are based on the so-called "visual inefficiency" hypothesis, so plausible because most of us do read visually (unless we are blind and we use Braille). None of these "visual efficiency" interventions carried out by optometrists have been found to be supported by any evidence, but they persist to this day because they seem so obvious, so plausible, in their appeal to parents and even to some teachers. Research has shown that reading has much less to do with imperfect vision or eye movements than with the several levels of the language system, starting with speech sounds. Certainly, visual acuity due to errors of refraction (near-sighted or far-sighted eyes) needs to be corrected by lenses in eyewear to permit the very entry level of reading; but when it comes to some of the other visual system components, less relevance is supported. In the "gray zone" of visual involvement would be dealing with convergence insufficiency, for which certain lenses can be provided so that the eyes are able to team up for converging and thus focusing. (The lenses of our eyes become too rigid to perform as we age and therefore need reading glasses, but in children the movements of convergence can be involved.) However, the eye movement therapies are completely without rationales in terms of the map of the brain. There are frontal eye fields for *scanning* stationary visual displays, making the movements we initiate, called "voluntary saccades" (rapid eye movements) that we use in reading. Many of the exercises for eye movements involve another eye movement system, initiated by the parietal eye fields pretty far away from the frontal eye fields, used for *tracking*, which means following with your eyes something that moves. It is this category of eye movements, tracking, that is the target of optometric eye exercises but is irrelevant to reading. (Tracking would be involved in hitting a baseball, shooting a flying bird, flying a kite, or any task dependent upon seeing and following movement. (I emphasize that we do not track movement when we read, except perhaps for the "crawl" on television newscasts, at the bottom or top of the screen.) Most of our reading depends upon the eye movements called scanning, making saccades of the voluntary variety. All of the exercises involving tracking are

providing an intervention to an eye movement system that is not used in reading. I have never seen anybody do an intervention exercise involving scanning, so there is little to report on whether or not that might have a positive impact on reading.

There was a brief interest in another vision therapy using colored overlays for reading, based on the idea that there were inefficiencies in a particular component of the visual system and remediated by filtering of the light, but there is no evidence for the efficacy of this intervention, nor is there consensus about the existence of the particular visual impairment in the majority of people with dyslexia.

7. Another kind of movement control thought to be related to reading became the object of interest of a group who thought that the cerebellum, so much concerned with all kinds of motor/procedural learning and ongoing governance of movement, could be involved in learning to read. This research group claimed to demonstrate cerebellar-based deficiencies in groups called "dyslexic," although strictly speaking the group studied was not sufficiently examined for us to know whether the members showed any other developmental problems in addition to dyslexia. (It is sometimes the case that when a problem is in the foreground but there are coexisting problems in the background, intervention will be aimed at the background factor; my somewhat facetious way of addressing this is by warning, "You can't turn blue eyes brown by dying hair brown.") The cerebellar-focused intervention prescribed consisted of remedial physical exercises enhancing postural stability and other supposedly cerebellar-based movements. The concept was that improvements in these movements were used to tune up the cerebellum to make that part of the brain support better learning of reading. This is an example of what we call a "process-focused intervention," which means that you are not going directly to intervene concerning reading but you are addressing a prerequisite to reading, structural or functional, improving brain processes essential as "platforms" for learning how to read. There is no evidence that this movement-based intervention focused on "tuning up" the cerebellum has resulted in improvements in acquisition of reading skill.

8. In general, "prerequisite training" or "process-focused" programs, many carried out by one school (but not all) of occupational

therapy, lack evidence for either relevance or efficacy. Occupational therapy remains popular because it appeals to parents and teachers with its child-friendly approaches and its promises for a relatively short duration of intervention that is claimed to result in permanent brain changes promoting school learning thereafter, very much like the cerebellar intervention described above.

More recently, our intoxication with using computerized educational programs was popularized and received a great deal of attention with a program that was called Fast ForWord (FFW) a computer program that was focused on basic auditory processing as a time-based capability. It was an elaborate program that was designed by some very high-level celebrated neuroscientists who felt that they could change the basic rapid temporal processing of auditory signals that would underlie both spoken and written language learning. It seemed to be coming from the best expertise derived from neuroscience and computer science. It promised a great deal, but it has not been documented to be uniquely or permanently effective and certainly did not replace interventions that deal directly with the reading skills themselves. There have been many articles claiming results gained in spoken language and in reading skill based on FFW, but there has not been any long-term independent, peer-reviewed, and well-controlled study supporting it. It is the most sophisticated of the prerequisite training, process-focused "fixes" assuming that reading will follow "as night follows day." Another computer program currently popular trains working memory, using exercises that are supposed to strengthen working memory in a fundamental way that generalizes to academic skills improvement.

9. I have discussed in another chapter the neuromyth of developmental risk factors for left-handers.

In summary, there is a great deal of interest in using knowledge about the brain to design educational practices in general and special interventions in particular, but many of them are based on incomplete or exaggerated extrapolations from neuroscience findings and have not been supported by independent peer-reviewed and well-controlled studies. They are largely based on the idea of intervention targets being underlying or antecedent processes that could be "fixed" or at least "tuned up" to improve a fundamental developmental platform for learning specific academic skills.

I felt strongly in my clinical years that one of the most important things I could do would be to steer parents away from these unsubstantiated but often very attractive interventions; children's time, their childhood, is not infinite, not to be wasted on ineffective interventions, and parents' wallets are not bottomless with respect to the expenditures for these interventions that are usually not "covered" by any form of insurance.

12

An Inconvenient Brain in the Context of Changes in Educational Environments

Since most children with "inconvenient brains" are those who have "disabilities" mild enough that we can assume they are able to survive educational challenges and live normal lives, the structure and offerings of the educational system that is their environment is obviously of great importance to outcomes. So in this last chapter, I will trace the history and current changes of American public education/special education over the past five decades, from my perspective as an advocate for children with "inconvenient brains."

When I first entered this field, both clinics and research concerned with children who needed some kind of special educational intervention, there were limited public education resources. Most of the special classes available within school systems were devoted to children with serious and obvious disabilities (blindness, deafness, cerebral palsy, intellectual limitations). Many children with dyslexia received privately funded help from paramedical professionals, through their parents' medical insurance; in the days when there were no such services offered within public school systems, parents could ask their pediatricians to prescribe "language therapy" by referral to a speech/language pathologist, whose services could include reading instruction. It was an established fact that many children with speech/language delays would also go on to experience reading problems, so it was a small step to remediate "language arts" with those who had "unexpected reading failure" even without a preschool speech/language delay. This professional perspective also made for sensitivity to and remediation for the word-finding difficulties of many children who are considered dyslexic, which to this day is recognized by some but not all experts on dyslexia. It was also a model for one-to-one ratio remediation, an expensive but, in my opinion, underestimated optimization of intervention for the most remediation-resistant poor readers. Many children did quite well with this private paramedical help, insurance-subsidized and maintained for their entire K-12 educational years. There also existed boarding schools devoted to integrating the remediation of dyslexia into their curriculum; these were expensive and entirely outside any medical insurance or educationally subsidized model, so only the wealthy were served in these often excellent facilities. (Some famous men were students at dyslexia-friendly boarding schools; some subsequently became advocates for special education for "learning disabilities" and financial donors to organizations devoted to this cause.)

Once there began to be state and federal laws mandating the provision of appropriate services for the large numbers of children with "learning disabilities" (and this long preceded any official recognition of school responsibility for children with ADHD, ASD, or any of the other less well-defined disabilities), medical insurance coverage vanished. Parents were told that services were now, by law, taken care of by and within the public education system. Even insurance-funded private speech/language or occupational therapy was limited to certain narrow circumstances, when the physical cause of the impairments existed; insurance forms began to require documentation as to whether the disability, the consequence of which was the school problem, was due to an illness or injury and the date of onset of that illness or injury. This meant that, like the boarding schools devoted to educating those with dyslexia, the private special services were available only to those who could afford such self-pay expenditures for many years.

As I stated in my introduction, I was fortunate to have started my acquaintance with public education and services dedicated to "inconvenient brains" in the state of New Jersey, where a law mandating special classes for the "neurologically impaired" preceded similar laws in many other states and the federal law. "Neurologically impaired" classes were recognizing the compatibility of normal intelligence with specific "intrinsic" academic deficiencies. Later, in other states in which I lived and worked, the "special needs" laws, using gentler language, combined with the federal mandate to create a series of services that were expressed as different levels of intensity of special education. There was a finely graded system of providing services that could range from progress monitoring through substantially separate placement in centers dedicated to the designated disability category; and with successful years in maximal levels of special education placement, there could be a de-escalation of services gradually returning the student to the minimal level, progress monitoring.

There were elaborate and often arcane ways of determining the eligibility of students for each of the disability categories, most often the academic skills deficit(s) being used for eligibility for provision of an Individualized Educational Plan (IEP) by the now skeptically regarded "discrepancy formula." In spite of the difficulties and inconsistencies introduced by some of the formulaic ways of determining eligibility, there was at least a period of time, about 20 years, between 1975 and 1995, when there existed in all of the states in which I have lived and worked (New Jersey, Massachusetts, and Maryland) a menu of options for appropriately remediating and also generally educating those with "inconvenient brains."

The first upheaval came in the middle of the 1990s, when, with the best of intentions, a consortium of parents and special educators began to promote greater *inclusion*. This was something different from "mainstreaming," which had meant that in one or more "good" subjects or in the course of decreasing levels of service (because of sufficient improvement in the subject in which the student was considered "learning disabled") the student would be a participant in the regular education classroom, perhaps with some modifications in the curriculum or the productivity requirements. Inclusion was a different philosophy; I must say that inclusion appears to have worked best for children with intellectual disabilities or even with sensory handicaps, but in my experience, it has not met its goals for those with "inconvenient brains."

The goals were that while academic progress was important, the ability to be integrated into the regular classroom and thus gain social skills necessary for ultimate adaptation to the world of work and community life would be achieved in best balance. For children with "inconvenient brains," however, often inclusion has meant receiving less in the way of time or intensity of special instruction; while socialization gains were not so obvious as was the case, for example, with the population that seemed to benefit the most from inclusion, children with Down's Syndrome. (One of the boys with dyslexia who came to my clinic said, "I wish I had some physical sign of my learning disability, so kids wouldn't be so mean to me or mock me for my not knowing stuff.")

The delivery of services in the regular classroom was less than adequate, even leaving aside the term optimal, because in the busy and usually somewhat noisy atmosphere of the classroom the special educator pulling up a chair to one or more students for a presumably remedial instruction session was a situation complicated by distraction or embarrassment.

Those who favored inclusion for the more mildly disabled student failed to recognize that being remediated within a room in full sight of your peers is just as embarrassing as being "pulled out" to go to a resource room or to attend school in an entirely different classroom. Those with the "inconvenient brains" are fully sensitive to how they look to others and how others are regarding them. The hope that inclusion would avoid stigmatization and therefore relative exclusion from the regular social community of peers has not been realized, while what has been sacrificed in large measure has been the efficacy of the remedial instruction. (I would add here that the other large group of children, those with ADHD, who have accommodations under a different law, rather than IEPs, or who may, because of their one-third overlap status as learning disabled also have IEPs, are similarly disadvantaged in the inclusion model, since they are most unlikely to resist attractive social opportunities in order to concentrate on studying in the regular classroom setting.) I am also skeptical that a child with ASD who has an aide in the regular classroom really has access to socialization with the typical children, unless some very sophisticated and imaginative approaches are implemented by the aide and the teacher.

Then we come to the twenty-first century, when more changes heap upon students more environmental stressors. These add to the disadvantages I refer to as the "inclusion delusion." We come to the age of "accountability" and "No Child Left Behind." This was an educational policy set forth with the greatest of idealism and good intentions (but we know where good intentions may lead) proposing that the "soft bigotry of low expectations" would be erased by holding every educational entity accountable by means of documenting whether there was sufficient annual improvement in the test scores of their students. This created an environment of anxiety at all levels of the educational environment and made particularly unrealistic demands that those who were in the categories of special education should also have to be included in the testing paradigm. All of this was done with minimal evidence that this kind of omnibus accountability would actually result in improved educational outcomes and with little sophistication about the methodology of testing (especially for those with "inconvenient brains") or the statistical analysis of longitudinal data. (For example, asking for improvement of test scores from schools already producing superior scores betrays lack of understanding of how little meaningful improvement at that high end would be possible, given the nature of the "bell shaped curve" of distribution of scores.)

I don't think I need to tell most readers of this book, whether they have read about it or because of their close association with students with "inconvenient brains," or if they are in any way involved with teaching and/or bringing up children, that the era of No Child Left Behind and the anxiogenic (anxiety provoking) environment that descended like dark clouds (or perhaps shrouds) upon the educators and the children alike in our public school systems was a major setback for education in the United States.

While the largely punitive frame of reference of "No Child Left Behind" gave way to the years of "Race to the Top," with its financial benefits to states contingent on implementation of certain policies (this was more of a positive reinforcement, de-emphasizing the punitive) the accountability philosophy persisted; then it reached its most problematic zenith with the promotion of and reward for the Common Core curriculum. (We have yet to see whether the revision of the NCLB law, ESSA (the Every Student Succeeds Act), and the less popular status of Common Core will make the atmosphere better.)

The Common Core curriculum and the tests which were designed to become its accountability metrics were devised by a group of people who employed the strategy of "back-mapping" from final high school graduation goals, desired attainments, or levels of competence in academic subjects. Including kindergarten in the 13 "chunks" of curriculum in each core academic subject, there was no attempt to be developmentally appropriate or to be aware of the nonlinear nature, year by year, of developmental windows of opportunity for learning. Representation by teachers of young children (the early years, 4–7) was token at best. The tests were put together in a manner that suggested ideals of acquisition of learning; the theoretical considerations outweighed any based upon developmental science, much less neuroscience.

Over the years, teachers concerned about the Common Core and the tests constructed to represent its standards managed to get to me samples of language arts and math tests. (Of course, this was a biased sample, since the teachers who wanted me to see these tests harbored questions or concerns about their appropriateness.) I must say, however, that these samples were usually several traditional grade levels in expectation above the actual grade levels of those taking the tests, and the design of the questions left a great deal to be desired in terms of the research on how to measure what you say you are measuring. (For example, reading comprehension items might have as the correct answer a statement that was not contained in the reading passage but would have to have been derived from outside knowledge.)

Simultaneous with and running alongside of the testing and accountability issues and the developmental insensitivity of the Common Core was a trend to declare, "Kindergarten is the new first grade." The rationale was often given that since most children attended some form of preschool, there was no need for kindergarten to continue to be a place to play and expand oral communication (language) skills. First came a push for getting involved in "phonological awareness" training, which was not bad in and of itself, but which became the driving force behind introducing the skill of phonics. Not only did kindergarten become more "academic" but the trend "back-mapped" itself into the four-year-old level. It became increasingly difficult to shop for toys for children without having some educational relevance prominently displayed or the content of the toy itself being emblazoned with letters of the alphabet, numerals, or shapes. The entire concept of academic "readiness" seemed to be abandoned in the rush to push children to acquire the academic skills of reading, writing (even more problematic), and arithmetic at an ever-earlier age, what I call pushing a "prematurization" of education. (By analogy to delivering a baby prematurely, the educational system can deliver curriculum prematurely!) Not only did the classes for four-year-olds and five-year-olds become overrun with academic tasks, but these displaced physical activity, play, having books read to the children and discussed, music, crafts, painting, and all of the other arts and involvements that, in a previous chapter, I have already pointed out as valuable in terms of actually promoting and enhancing learning and/or underlying brain development. The "prematurization of formal education" also increased the risk that children not *developmentally ready* for academic skills would be included among the "learning disabled," thus unnecessarily swelling the ranks of those needing services (already underfunded and inadequate for those whose "inconvenient brains" genuinely need help) and putting up a wall of frustration for those simply not ready. The unnecessarily frustrated academically "unready" children are likely to make life decisions that they and school are not meant for each other, with far-reaching emotional consequences.

The accountability philosophy also came to be accompanied by a bipartisan commitment to the idea of "school reform" toward the goal of raising test scores, a large part of which is expressed in "school choice." In practical terms, this meant the proliferation of charter schools. Now, the charter school idea arose itself from teachers and the leaders of teachers' unions, with the idea that these would not be for profit but would be model schools within public school systems, serving as innovative educational "laboratories" from which successful programs could be scaled up and generalized to the public school system in which the charter school resided. This is still true in a minority of cases. More and more data is accumulating, however, that seems to point to the fact that most charter schools are not doing any better than the public schools from which they are taking financial resources. For-profit charters have become prominent in many states. Little supervision or oversight is demanded for charter schools. (This seems odd in an era in which "accountability" in terms of students, teachers, and principals in the public schools is so widely demanded.) Many charter schools are privately managed but publicly funded, so that they are "public" in name only.

Charter schools have been particularly lacking in proper responses to children with "inconvenient brains." It is beyond the scope of this chapter or this book to go into all of the problems presented in this regard by charter schools, which have claimed misleading statistics touting successes, such as not counting attrition when calculating percentages who get desired test scores or graduate from high school, or not allowing refilling of slots past a certain mid-elementary school level so as to keep the "denominator" of those who are to be counted as successful within the control of the charter school. In addition, charter schools have frequently suffered financial mismanagement, financial fraud, sudden closures in the middle of school years, high teacher turnover due to regimentation, work overloads, and lack of reasonable workplace safety, all happening in the unregulated charter systems.

This book is focused upon children with "inconvenient brains," and for them the charter school movement has been largely a further stressor. Many such children are "bounced back" to their parent public schools, where the draining of resources towards the charter schools has made funding for the needed special education services even leaner.

As I have said, a great deal of this school reform as expressed through school choice has been politically bipartisan, rhetorically eloquent, and motivated by good intentions. The point is that talking appealingly about education and feeling good intentions about education are no substitutes for having some knowledge of children's development, in the broader sense of the word that includes neurological development, and having some evidence-based reasons to construct curriculum or to construct and depend upon tests for accountability. The broader purpose of public education has been to provide opportunities for the "pursuit of happiness," participation as citizens, and optimal life adaptations. This idealistic goal coupled with the ever-expanding knowledge of the nature of those for whom we are providing the opportunities would seem to be imperative if we are to get back on track in the educational environment of the United States, not only for those with "inconvenient brains," but for all children. In many ways, there is very little in terms of educational needs that distinguishes children from disadvantaged backgrounds from children who, despite the highest level of advantage, happen to be born with "inconvenient brains."

> Positivity is of overarching importance, as a principle of reinforcement in behavior modification, as a general background attitude towards children, and as a design to balance experiences of strengths with those of weaknesses characteristic of "the inconvenient brain."
>
> ("You've got to emphasize the positive, eliminate the negative, latch on to the affirmative…")

For all students, the basic background of education should not be anxiogenic, it should be one of positively oriented shaping of learning and behavior, with an encouraging and enabling attitude.

Among students, there is a great deal of diversity of every kind, of which "the inconvenient brain" is only one example, what some like to call "neurodiversity." A public education system cannot be so narrow in terms of its standards and values (test score accountability) nor so purely theoretical in its commitment to concepts like "choice" without collecting sufficient documentation and evidence to support and implement such important decision-making.

References

Brain Development and Other General Information

- Aamodt, S. and Wang, S. *Welcome to Your Child's Brain.* Bloomsbury, USA, New York, 2011.
- Lieberman, M.D. *Social: Why Our Brains Are Wired to Connect.* Crown Publishers, New York, 2013.

Executive Function

- Meltzer, L. (editor) *Executive Function in Education: From Theory to Practice,* Second Edition. The Guilford Press, New York and London, 2018.

Autistic Spectrum Disorder

- Grandin, T. *The Autistic Brain: Helping Different Kinds of Minds Succeed.* Mariner Books, New York, 2014.
- Myers, J.M. *How to Teach Life Skills to Kids with Autism or Asperger's.* Future Horizons, Arlington, TX, 2010.
- Robison, J.E. *Be Different: My Adventures with Asperger's and My Advice for Fellow Aspergians, Misfits, Families and Teachers.* Broadway Books, New York, 2012.

Attention Deficit Hyperactivity Disorder

- Barkley, R.M. *Attention Deficit Hyperactivity Disorder*, Fourth Edition. The Guilford Press, New York and London, 2015.
- Nigg, J.T. *Getting Ahead of ADHD*. The Guilford Press, New York and London, 2017.

Dyslexia

- Shaywitz, S. *Overcoming Dyslexia*. Random House, New York, 2005 (New title edition).
- Wolf, M. *Proust and the Squid*. Harper Perennial, New York, 2008 (Reprint edition).

Learning Disabilities

- Fletcher, J.M., Lyon, G.R., Fuchs, L.S., Barnes, M.A. (editors). *Learning Disabilities: From Identification to Intervention*. Second Edition, The Guilford Press, New York and London, 2018.

Websites

- Autistic Self-Advocacy Network (http://autisticadvocacy.org)
- Children's National Hospital (https://childrensnational.org) (look for Autism or ASD Parent Guide)
- Kennedy Krieger Institute (Center for Autism and Related Disorders) (https://kennedykrieger.org)
- CHADD (Children with Hyperactive & Attention Deficit Disorders) (www.chadd.org)
- IDA (International Dyslexia Association) (https://dyslexiaida.org/)
- LDA (Learning Disabilities Association) (www.understood.org)

Index

Page numbers in *italics* denote figures.

academic over-emphasis in early learning 118–119
accountability and testing 116–119, 120
Adderall 69
ADHD (attention deficit hyperactivity disorder) 16, 58; co-occurrence with ASD 66–67; and DCD 41–42, 72; diagnosis of 72, 76, 80; and EDF 46–47, 75–77, 78, 80; and gender 80; history of 69–73; and inclusion model of education 116; and learning disabilities 101; neurological aspects 70, 71–72, 74–76; and NVLD 98; and play 19, 60–61; and SLI 28; and social exclusion 80–81; stimulant medications 69, 72–73, 78–79, 81–82; sugar consumption not implicated 106; and Tourette Syndrome 40, 76; treatment programs 80, 81, 82
adolescence 14–15, 18, 65; and self-control mechanisms 106–107; and SLI 30
algebra 29, 96
alphabetic principle 55, 85–86, 92
alternative treatments, discredited and revived 5
American Board of Psychiatry and Neurology 1
amygdala (emotional brain) 15, 17, 50
animals and number sense 94–95
anxiety and EDF 50, 75, 78, 82
aphasia 2, 71, 89
arithmetic 24, 29, 51–52, 67, 95–96, 99–100

art-infused education 21
artistic ability and fine motor coordination 38
ASD (Autistic Spectrum Disorder): and ADHD 66–67; and Asperger Syndrome 54–55; aversion to change 61; causes of 64, 68n1; child's relationship with parents 60, 61; communication impairment 57–58; diagnosis of 56, 60, 63–65, 68; and inclusion model of education 67, 116; interventions and prognosis 66–67; lack of empathy 59; language impairment 24, 31; learning and memory 55, 67; play 60–61, 62; sensory stimuli 63; and social skills 59–60
Asperger, Dr. Hans 54, 55, 58
Asperger Syndrome: in adults 62–63; and education 67; and high functioning autism 54–56, 61; and play 62
athletics 21, 22, 33, 37, 40
Attention Deficit Disorder 71, 74
auditory processing 26, 27–28, 58, 67, 89–90, 111
auditory stimuli 10–11, 20–21
author's CV 1–5
axons 10, 11–12

Barkley, Dr. Russell 81
behavior regulation 43, 51, 101, 107; and play 18–19
behavioral management therapy 80, 82
behaviors: disruptive 73–74;

behaviors *continued*
  inappropriate 56, 60, 67; restricted repetitive repertoire in ASD 56, 57, 63
bilingualism 19–20, 21
boarding schools and dyslexia 114
Boston Naming Test 87
Broca's area 88, 89

cerebellum 45, 110
cerebral cortex 9, 10, 11, 36, 97; and ADHD 74; and language 19–20
cerebral palsy 71, 89
charter schools 119–120
chess 62
chimpanzees and numbers 94–95
Chinese language 19–20, 86, 91
circadian rhythms in teenagers 18
cognitive control 43–44, 45–46, 72; and ADHD 73–76, 80; *see also* EF (executive function)
Common Core curriculum 117–118
comprehension and reading 28–29, 51, 92, 100–101, 118; and language 14, 111
connections in the brain 10–15, 19; and EF 48–49; and language 88–89; and mathematics 99; *see also* myelination in brain development
cool executive function *see* cognitive control
corpus callosum 14, 15
critical periods in learning 12, 15

DCD (Developmental Coordination Disorder) 33, 34, 37, 40–41, 72
decoding skills and reading 28, 86, 88–89, 93, 100–101
dendrites 10, 12, 104
'disabilities' and 'disorders' official but unsuitable terms 7
disability and educational resources 63, 82, 113–116
distraction 50, 79
D (M)CD (Developmental (Motor) Coordination Disorder) 28, 100
Double Deficit scheme of dyslexia 91

Down Syndrome 24, 115
DSM-5 (*Diagnostic and Statistical Manual*) 7, 33; ADHD and ASD dual diagnosis 66; and behavior 57; does not recognize Asperger Syndrome 54, 56; specific reading disability 85
dyscalculia 2, 99
dysgraphia 89, 100
dyslexia 16, 24, 27, 83, 100–101; boarding schools 114; characteristics of 85–87; diagnosis of 90–91; and EDF 50; insurance and costly remediation interventions 113–114; intervention programs 92–93; neurological aspects 87–89; reversals in reading and writing not a factor 107–108; and SLI 26, 27, 28; visual inefficiency hypothesis interventions 109–110
dyspraxia 33–34

Early Infantile Autism 55
EDF (executive dysfunction) 44–45, 52–53; and ADHD 46–47, 75–77, 78, 80; and anxiety 50
EF (executive function) 75–76, 100–101; analogies for 47; dependence on neural connections *48*; developmental stages of 43–46, *44*, 49; general core skills relating to 47–48; and inhibition 79, 81; in MLD and NVLD 96–98; testing of 77–78
eligibility for special educational needs 115
emotion and learning 15–16, 21–22
emotional control 19, 43, 45–46, 73–74, 75, 80; in teenagers 106–107
emotional expression 81
emotional prosody 90
empathy 19, 59
English language irregularities 85, 92

environmental influences on child development 6, 15, 49, 52, 104; and ADHD 71, 72
ESSA (Every Student Succeeds Act) 117
exploration 46, 49; aversion to in ASD children 60–61
expressive language impairment 27, 28–30, 87–88
extracurricular activities in schools 21–22, 37, 118
eye movements and reading 109–110

Federal legislation 79, 114
FFW (Fast ForWord) computer educational program 111
fine motor coordination difficulties 33, 34–36, 37–38
foreign language learning 55, 86
frontal lobe 15, 20, 45, 59, 106, 107
frontal lobe syndrome and ADHD 75–76

games of chance and ASD 62
gender differences in brain development 12–13; and ADHD 80
general motor coordination problems and sports 37
generalization, inability for children with ASD 67–68
geometry 96
Geschwind, Norman 1, 3
glia 10, 11
goal-oriented mental processes 43–44
good enough for life levels of development 29, 45, 74
gray matter (neurons, brain cells) 20
Gross, Carol 81
gross motor coordination difficulties 33–34, 37

handwriting and motor coordination problems 32–35, 38–39, 40
hearing impairment and SLI 23
hemispheres of the brain 13; and arithmetic 100; and auditory processing 90; and bilingualism 19–20; *corpus callosum* connections 14, 15; enhanced integration through musical training 21; and language skills 14, 16; learning styles myth 105–106; left side and SLI 24, 27, 28; MLD and NVLD 97–98, 99
higher order mental processes 14, 26, 34, 43–44, 89
hippocampus 13
homework 33
hot executive function *see* social-emotional control

IEPs (Individualized Educational Plans) 79, 115, 116
immunization and ASD 65–66
inclusion in mainstream education, inadequacies of 5–6, 79, 115–116
Inconvenient Brain, genesis of the term 6–7
inhibition 43–44, 46, 49; and ADHD 78–79, 81; essential for attention in education 50, 79
inhibitory control, factors impeding development of 52
instinctual behavior 19, 61
IQ (intelligence quotient): and dyslexia 85, 87, 90–91; and LD 102; nonverbal and SLI 28, 30; testing and EF 49

Johns Hopkins University 1, 55, 64
joint attention, lack of in ASD 60, 61

K-12 (kindergarten to twelfth grade) education 6; and myelination 12
Kanner, Dr. Leo 55, 64
Kennedy Krieger Institute 1
keyboard skills 39, 40
kindergarten and Common Core curriculum 117, 118–119

kittens' development through play 19

language, levels of 25–26, *25*, 83–84, *84*
language circuit of the brain 88
language skills 13–14, 25, 56, 58, 111; and ADHD 77; and early development 23; *see also* bilingualism; SLI (Specific Language Impairment)
language therapy 30, 113
late blooming in boys' development 12, 14
late talkers 29–30
LD (learning disability), diagnosis and intervention 71, 79–80, 81, 102–103
learning and memory 55, 85–86, 95–96; importance of sleep 18
left-handedness 13, 16, 88
legislation and learning disabilities 114–115
long division and executive function 96

marshmallow test 46
mathematics 21, 51–52, 94; and language impairment 24, 29; *see also* MLD (mathematics learning disability)
measles 65–66
medical insurance and learning disabilities 113–114
memory, different kinds of 13, 55; *see also* learning and memory; working memory
metacognition 44
Minimal Brain Dysfunction 69, 70–72
MLD (mathematics learning disability) 95–96, 97–98; numbers and language 99
motor control: and ADHD 41, 72, 74; and EF 45; and writing 34–36
motor coordination and musical instrument playing 38, 39–40
motor coordination development 3, 74, 78

motor skills learning, retention of 36
mouth position and speech sounds 26, 27, 89
MRI (magnetic resonance imaging): and ADHD 74; and ASD diagnosis 64–65; and language impairment 24–25, 27, 56
musical training, benefits of 20–21, 39–40
myelination in brain development 11–12, 14, 15; and handwriting problems 35, 36; and motor development 42

NCLB (No Child Left Behind) law 116–117
neural axon-dendrite connections 10–11
neurodiversity 6, 121
neuroeducation 4, 104
neuroimaging 9
neurons 9, 10, 12, 20, 49, 51
neuroplasticity 20
neuropsychology 1–2, 55, 97–98
neuroscience and educational practice 18, 100, 103, 104, 106, 111–112
neurotransmitters 25, 50, 75
New Jersey state laws and the neurologically impaired 70, 71, 114
NINDS (National Institute of Neurological Diseases and Stroke) 70
noise and ASD 63
nonright-handedness 13, 16, 88, 90
nonverbal cognition 27, 28, 105
nonverbal communication 57, 58, 65
numbers and language 29, 95, 99
nurture and brain development 10
NVLD (nonverbal learning disability) 97, 98, 99

occupational therapy 110–111; and motor coordination 36, 41
Orton, Dr. Samuel Torrey on visual reversals 107–108

OTMP (organization, time management and planning) coaching 79, 80
overflow movements as neurodevelopmental anomalies 72, *73*

PANESS (Physical and Neurological Examination for Subtle Signs) 42
peer group exclusion 29, 37, 62, 80–81, 116
pencil grasp in children learning to write 34–37, *35*, 38
phonemes 26, 89
phonology *see* speech sounds
picture naming tests 86–87
planum temporale 27, 90
play, role in learning and development 18–19, 118–119
positivity and behavior modification 120
postnatal brain development 11–12
postural instability in handwriting problems 40
Prechtl Choreiform Syndrome and handwriting 40
prefrontal cortex 75–76
prematurization of education 118–119
prenatal brain development 9, 10–11
printing and cursive handwriting 36, 38–39
problem-solving 17, 46; and working memory 51–52
procedural learning 13, 55, 110; and writing 34–36
process-focused intervention programs 110–111
processing speed 27–28, 49, 50–51, 100, 101
prosody in vocal tone 57
pruning in brain development 11, 12; in adolescence 14–15
psychoanalysis 64
puberty 12, 13, 65

RAN (Rapid Automatized Naming) test 3, *91*

reading comprehension 28–29, 51, 85–86, 88, 100–101, 118
reading remediation techniques 92–93
reversals in reading and writing 107–109
Ritalin 69, 73
Rourke, Dr. Byron P. 97
RTI (Response to Intervention) and learning disabilities 102–103
Rudel, Dr. Rita G. 2–3, 107

school reform 119, 120–121
self-control 81, 106–107
self-monitoring 15, 44, 97, 101
semantics 25, 26, 83, *84*, 85, 87, 88–89
sleep 17–18
SLI (Specific Language Impairment): and dyslexia 27; and schooling 28–29, 30, 31; and social competence 29–30; and speech sounds 27–28
social interaction, impairments in 57–58, 60, 61
social learning deprivation 66
social-emotional control 45–46, 81; and ADHD 73–74, 75–76, 80; development of in teenagers 106–107
socialization and SLI 29–30
Specific Learning Disability, definition of 70–71
specific reading disability 84–85
speech sounds 25–28; and dyslexia 83–84, 86–87, 88–89, 90
spelling 85, 89, 92, 100, 107
sports activities and DCD 37, 40–41
stimulant medication and ADHD 69, 72–73, 78–79, 81–82
strephosymbolia 108
strokes and cognitive deficits 2, 3, 85, 89, 98
subitizing 94, 99
sugar and hyperactivity 106
synapses 10; networks developed 11, 12

teaching children with ASD 67–68

team sports contra-indicated by DCD 40–41
teasing 59
testing and special educational needs 116–119
Theory of Mind 59
Tourette Syndrome 40, 76

visual arts 21, 22
visual inefficiency hypothesis not a factor in dyslexia 109
visual-motor coordination 34, 38–39
visual-spatial ability and mathematics 95–97, 99

Voeller, Dr. Kytja 98

Wernicke's area 88
white matter (connections) 11, 20
Wing, Dr. Lorna and Asperger Syndrome 54, 55
Wolf, Marianne and dyslexia 91
word memorization 85–86
word retrieval difficulties 29, 87, 96
working memory 43, 49, 50–52, 100; and numbers 94–95, 96–97; reading comprehension 101, 111; and speech sounds 27